Addiction and Recovery in the U

Addiction and Recovery in the UK captures the essence of the emerging addictions recovery movement and in particular the emerging evidence base that had been gathered around the umbrella of the Recovery Academy UK. The Recovery Academy was established with the aim of creating a forum for people in recovery, practitioners, commissioners and academics working together to describe and understand the principles of recovery as applied across the UK. Following the first annual conference, researchers who had been involved in academic research on recovery and innovative services and activities that had been evaluated were invited to outline UK initiatives. This book, the result of their contributions, is a vibrant collection of diverse theories and models, critiques and innovations, ranging from two linked papers describing the growing recovery movement in Edinburgh to a recovery walking group in Wales and a model for peer activities in the North of England. The projects are typically 'community up' projects whose essence has been captured within this book, and which together paint a picture of vitality and growth in the UK recovery movement.

This book was originally published as a special issue of the *Journal of Groups in Addiction and Recovery*.

Jeffrey D. Roth, MD, FASAM, FAGPA is the medical director of Working Sobriety Chicago, an outpatient treatment program for addiction in the USA. He is editor-in-chief of the *Journal of Groups in Addiction and Recovery* and author of *Group Psychotherapy and Recovery from Addiction: Carrying the Message* (2004).

David Best is Associate Professor of Addiction Studies at Monash University and Turning Point Alcohol and Drug Centre in Melbourne, Australia. He works in the areas of recovery research and treatment effectiveness and is a Chartered Psychologist and Criminologist.

David Bryce was the founder member of Calton Athletic Recovery Group, established in 1985 as a direct result of David's own experience of addiction and recovery. A tireless and passionate campaigner for recovery, he dedicated his time and energy to supporting individuals into recovery through a programme of physical activity and mutual support. As a result, thousands of men and women have been given an opportunity to recover from drug and alcohol addiction. David's unshakeable belief in recovery and his determined pursuit of that goal in the face of reluctance and scepticism in mainstream treatment, brought hope and encouragement to families and communities far beyond his native Glasgow. Sadly, David is no longer with us, but his legacy lives on through the continuing work of Calton Athletic Recovery Group.

This book is dedicated to him.

Addiction and Recovery in the UK

Edited by
Jeffrey D. Roth and David Best

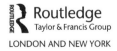
Routledge
Taylor & Francis Group

LONDON AND NEW YORK

First published 2013
by Routledge
2 Park Square, Milton Park, Abingdon, Oxfordshire OX14 4RN

Simultaneously published in the USA and Canada
by Routledge
711 Third Avenue, New York, NY 10017

First issued in paperback 2015

Routledge is an imprint of the Taylor & Francis Group, an informa business

British Library Cataloguing in Publication Data
A catalogue record for this book is available from the British Library

ISBN 13: 978-1-138-94675-0 (pbk)
ISBN 13: 978-0-415-63130-3 (hbk)

Typeset in Garamond
by Taylor & Francis Books

Publisher's Note
The publisher would like to make readers aware that the chapters in this book may be referred to as articles as they are identical to the articles published in the special issue. The publisher accepts responsibility for any inconsistencies that may have arisen in the course of preparing this volume for print.

Contents

Citation Information

The following chapters were originally published in the *Journal of Groups in Addiction and Recovery*, volume 6, issues 1-2 (2011). When citing this material, please use the original page numbering for each article, as follows:

Foreword
The Emerging UK Recovery Movement
William L. White
Journal of Groups in Addiction and Recovery, volume 6, issues 1-2 (2011) pp. 5-6

Chapter 2
Recovery and Public Policy: Driving the Strategy by Raising Political Awareness
David Best and Grace Ball
Journal of Groups in Addiction and Recovery, volume 6, issues 1-2 (2011) pp. 7-19

Chapter 3
The Evolution of a UK Evidence Base for Substance Misuse Recovery
Teodora Groshkova and David Best
Journal of Groups in Addiction and Recovery, volume 6, issues 1-2 (2011) pp. 20-37

Chapter 4
A Discussion of the Origins of The Road to Recovery – the Scottish Government's Recovery Policy for Drugs
Ria Din
Journal of Groups in Addiction and Recovery, volume 6, issues 1-2 (2011) pp. 38-48

Chapter 5
North West Recovery Forum: Recovery and Harm Reduction, the Odd Couple of Drug Treatment?
Mark Gilman and Rowdy Yates
Journal of Groups in Addiction and Recovery, volume 6, issues 1-2 (2011) pp. 49-59

Chapter 6
LEAP and the Recovery Community in Edinburgh
David McCartney
Journal of Groups in Addiction and Recovery, volume 6, issues 1-2 (2011) pp. 60-75

Notes on Contributors

Matt Baker is a qualified Teacher and Outdoor Instructor who has previously worked with a number of client groups including teenagers with Learning Disabilities, children with Autistic Spectrum Disorders and people with Psychosis. A strong believer in client centred approaches that support the individual to achieve lasting change, he spent several years working for the Drug Intervention Programme before co-creating an experimental intervention aimed at clients with substance misuse history. This drew on the experiences of the group detailed in this article, utilising outdoor activities as a vehicle for delivering a therapeutic programme. Winner of a number of awards including the British Psychological Society student writing competition (2010) and the Bruner prize for Social Psychology (2011), Matt has recently completed a degree in psychology and is now training as an Educational Psychologist.

Grace Ball has worked in and around the addictions field for more than 20 years in various guises whilst achieving a degree in Health Science and a leadership qualification. Grace has a strong desire to see Recovery reflected in the local services provided for people with alcohol and other drug problems and is currently supporting a strategic redesign based on an integrated Recovery Oriented System of care model. Grace's PhD is looking at how to measure drug and alcohol professional worker attitudes towards Recovery and the impact these attitudes have on client groups. In addition, Grace has the role of Honorary Board Secretary for the Recovery Academy CIC managing all the RA business, leads on the organisation of the Recovery Academy Annual conference, the Recovery Champion awards and maintains an informal RA Membership list.

David Best is Associate Professor in Addiction Studies at Turning Point Alcohol and Drug Centre and Monash University in Melbourne. He leads the clinical research area and is strategic lead for higher education. David is qualified as a psychologist and criminologist, having studied at Strathclyde University and London School of Economics, and having been trained at the Institute of Psychiatry and Maudsley Hospital in London. Academically, he has also worked in the addictions research area at Strathclyde University, Birmingham University and the University of the West of Scotland. Additionally, he has worked on secondment at the National Treatment Agency for Substance Use and the Prime Minister's Delivery Unit. His research interests are in developing an evidence base around recovery and in implementing recovery-oriented systems of care. He has published over 100 research papers and is the author of two books on addiction recovery.

Ruth Campbell is Chief Executive of Comas, the community development agency supporting the development of the Serenity Café. Ruth has over 20 years of experience in community development and social inclusion, including stints in policy within central government and management in local government, providing a rounded view of the challenges facing recovery communities. She is a Clore Social Leadership Fellow.

Ria Din celebrates 25 years in working in addictions and recovery this year. In that time she has worked all over Scotland for local councils, the NHS, Third Sector organisations and the Scottish Government. Ria is proud to say that she realises she has learned everything she knows about addictions and recovery from those in recovery themselves. Ria spent five years at the Drug Policy Unit in the Scottish Government and feels privileged to have been involved in introducing a paradigm change in policy by being involved in writing the Road to Recovery and in helping set up the Scottish Recovery Consortium. Ria currently works for South Lanarkshire Council. She is a social worker with an M.A. (Hons) in Politics, a Masters in Social Work and a PG Cert in Addictions from what is now the University of the West of Scotland. She can be contacted at sorayadin@aol.com

Kane Duffy is a volunteer in recovery with the Serenity Café and a student of psychology at Heriot Watt University.

Michael Gaughan is a volunteer in recovery with the Serenity Café and works in hospital theatre support services and has been active in helping establish CA (Cocaine Anonymous) in Edinburgh.

Michael Mochrie is a volunteer in recovery with the Serenity Café.

Mark Gilman is the Strategic Recovery Lead for the National Treatment Agency for Substance Misuse in England. Mark is currently working on models for the coproduction of recovery that can work within a Public Health approach. Mark has a first degree in Organisation Theory and a MA in the study of Drugs, Crime and Social Deviance. Mark has been working with problem drug users since the 1970s. The creation of recovery communities is the primary purpose and recovery is about regeneration. We need to regenerate people as well as places. Recovery is a bridge to normal living for some of the most marginalised people. Mark Gilman is a committed friend and student of recovery. Mark's interest in the co-production of recovery is rooted in the optimism and hope that comes from joining with others to find common solutions to problems that seemed insurmountable as individuals.

Teodora Groshkova qualified with a first class honours in psychology, a Masters with merit in Clinical and Public Health Aspects of Addiction and a PhD in the Psychology of Addiction. She has worked as a researcher at the National Addiction Centre at King's College London before joining the European Monitoring Centre for Drugs and Drug Addiction in November 2010 as a scientific analyst focusing on health and social responses to addiction.

Sidney Jobber was born in London in 1955. His parents moved to Ellesmere Port Cheshire when he was two years old, where he grew up with two brothers and two sisters, all being educated at Our Lady's Catholic Schools. In 1970 Sidney enlisted in the British Army joining the junior leaders Regiment for two years, and then the Cheshire Regiment. He saw active service in Belfast in 1974. After completing his army service, his main career was at Shell Chemicals Cheshire for 20 years as a process technician. He got married in 1979 and now has two wonderful daughters, and six grandchildren. After leaving Shell through redundancy he admitted himself to a rehabilitation unit in North Wales to deal with the alcohol problem he had acquired over the years. With a group of friends in recovery he started a walking mountaineering group, going on regular walks in the Snowdonia mountain range. The group then grew and became constituted and known as D.A.R.E. Sidney spent 2 years at Bangor University doing Sociology and is now hoping to study a substance misuse degree course.

Matt Kidd is an expert by experience who has been part of the recovery community in the North-West of England for a number of years and who is involved in the peer programme UChooseIt. Matt is a founding board member of the Recovery Academy in the UK.

Wulf Livingston currently works as a Senior Lecturer in Social Work at Glyndwr University. Prior to academia he worked in a range of community social work settings both voluntary and statutory, working predominantly in the field of alcohol and drugs. Wulf is nearing the completion of his qualitative PhD studies, exploring the acquisition of alcohol knowledge by social workers. His areas of research and publication interest are alcohol and drugs in social work, service user involvement and recovery. He continues to be an active member of a number of charities and organizations involved in either specific alcohol and drug research issues or community based recovery agendas. Prior to social care work, Wulf spent time in the catering industry and directly learning about drug and alcohol use.

Marion Logan is the Chief Executive of Phoenix Futures in Scotland. Marion is an experienced trainer and manager who has worked in the AOD field in both Scotland and England and has been a driver for the recovery movement in Scotland.

Margaret Malloch is a Senior Research Fellow with the Scottish Centre for Crime and Justice Research at the University of Stirling. She has extensive experience of conducting research in the field of addiction and recovery in Scotland, particularly in relation to criminal justice interventions for substance users. She has a specific interest in the ways in which social structures can impact upon individual experiences of recovery, particularly in relation to gender, class and ethnicity; and the ways in which 'grass-root' movements attempt to resist this influence.

David McCartney is currently the Clinical Lead at Lothians & Edinburgh Abstinence Programme, a partnership NHS/Council/NGO sector project for clients living in the Lothian area. David's background is in inner-city general practice in Glasgow. Following retraining in addictions he now works exclusively as a Primary Care Addiction Specialist in clinical and management roles. Previously a tutor on the Royal College of General Practitioners' Substance Misuse Management course, he has a Master's degree with distinction in Alcohol and Drug Studies. He enjoys teaching patients, medical and postgraduate students and primary care practitioners on the subjects of addiction and recovery. David is a member of the Royal College of General Practitioners. He is also a member of the Drugs Strategy Delivery Commission in Scotland, sits on the Government's Drug and Alcohol Delivery Group and is a Fellow of the RSA.

William White, MA, is a Senior Research Consultant at Chestnut Health Systems, past chair of the board of Recovery Communities United and a volunteer consultant with Faces and Voices of Recovery since its inception in 2001. He has authored or co-authored more than 300 addiction-related articles and monographs and 16 books, including *Slaying the Dragon: The History of Addiction Treatment and Recovery*.

Rowdy Yates is Senior Research Fellow and facilitator of Scottish Addiction Studies, University of Stirling. In 1971 he was co-founder of the Lifeline Project; one of the UK's longest established drug specialist services. He was co-editor of *Therapeutic Communities for the Treatment of Drug Users* and of *Tackling Addiction: Pathways to Recovery*. In 1994 he was awarded the MBE for services to the prevention of drug addiction. He is Director of the European Working Group on Drugs Oriented Research; Acting President of the European Federation of Therapeutic Communities); and Chair of the UK Recovery Academy.

FOREWORD

Since its inception in 2006, the *Journal of Groups in Addiction & Recovery* (*JGAR*) has ably addressed a broad spectrum of issues related to group and family work in addiction treatment, group approaches to the treatment of special populations (e.g., women, people with co-occurring disorders), and the influence of face-to-face and Internet-based recovery mutual aid societies and other recovery support institutions (e.g., recovery schools) on long-term recovery outcomes. This latest special issue of *JGAR* continues and extends that tradition by exploring an emerging and quite vibrant "recovery movement" in the United Kingdom.

The full import of the articles in this special issue is seen only when looking at them as a whole. They reveal a critical shift from pathology-based and intervention-based knowledge as the organizing centers of policy and service activity to knowledge drawn from the lived experience of long-term addiction recovery. The lessons being extracted from those collective recovery experiences are transforming social policies and clinical interventions, expanding and diversifying recovery mutual aid societies and new recovery support institutions, and mobilizing recovering individuals and families in such areas as policy advocacy, peer-based recovery support, and community service. This shift in emphasis is also setting the stage, through the newly formed Recovery Academy, for a recovery-focused research agenda and new structures for scientific inquiry and recovery-focused professional and community education.

The articles that follow offer deep insights into the history of the UK recovery movement and the contextual influences that set the stage for and continue to influence this movement. They provide insider accounts of everything from new recovery-focused policy formulation to the development of new recovery support organizations and services. But more than anything else, these articles convey the profound optimism and celebration that are at the heart of successful recovery movements.

A day is rapidly approaching when those seeking recovery in the United Kingdom will be attracted and welcomed by local cultures of recovery that will stand as living proof of the transformative power of recovery. A day is coming when these cultures will provide the psychological and social space within which people can achieve successful recovery initiation, recovery maintenance, and an enhanced quality of personal and family life in long-term recovery, and then be challenged to support others similarly affected. A day is rapidly coming in the United Kingdom when people who were once defined as the problem will have become an important and visible part of the solution. A day is coming when recovery movements will spread around the globe. When that day comes, historians will want to reconstruct how that day arrived. When they do, they will discover key elements of this early story in the following articles.

William L. White
Senior Research Consultant
Chestnut Health Systems, Punta Gorda, Florida, USA

Carrying the Message of Recovery across Political Boundaries

The Third Step of the Twelve Step Programs describes surrendering "to God as we understood Him." Whether or not Twelve Step Programs are seen as useful in recovery from addiction, clearly, recovery requires surrender to something other than the drug or process that defines the addiction. Finding a path that is different from the path of addiction is therefore central to the process of recovery. For such a path to have sufficient appeal to the addict, the signs on the path need to be written in a language accessible to the addict. The language of the Twelve Step Programs, born and raised in the United States, may have language, and therefore ideas, that seem foreign outside of the United States.

A popular joke describes the United States and the United Kingdom as two nations separated by a common language. In this special issue, we are pleased to offer evidence of the bridge that is being created by the Recovery Academy, a group of researchers and clinicians in the United Kingdom who are working on developing a model of recovery that will meet the needs of addicts in that nation. The Recovery Academy is headed by David Best, who has contributed several articles to previous issues of this journal, including our last issue on international perspectives on recovery from addiction. The Recovery Academy has also made extensive use of William White as a consultant to their process, and we are grateful to him for writing the introduction to this special issue and for his past contributions to the *Journal of Groups in Addiction and Recovery*.

The first half of this special issue examines the impact of public policy on recovery from addiction. Public policy affects the largest of our groups: the social system. Best and Ball describe the development of a recovery orientation toward the treatment of addiction in England and Scotland. Their description explicitly invites us to discover the transmission of recovery values in both directions across the Atlantic Ocean.

The next article, by Groshkova and Best, provides the evidence base for the recovery perspective that is developing in the United Kingdom. Their evidence is drawn from treatment outcomes and cohort studies. We may be reassured that the movement toward an evidence-based treatment paradigm is being pursued internationally.

The Recovery Academy is composed of colleagues who are not culturally homogeneous. Din writes about the experience of the Scottish Government in moving from goals that were primarily geared toward harm reduction to recovery-oriented goals. One particularly moving element of this transition is that it required the presence of a sufficient number of addicts in recovery to make this goal plausible.

Significantly, the movement in the United Kingdom toward a recovery orientation has not involved the abandonment of a harm reduction perspective. As illustrated by the inaugural issue of the *Journal of Groups in Addiction and Recovery*, the dichotomization of recovery and harm reduction has handicapped our ability to use the best of each perspective. The article by Gilman and Yates makes a case for the integration of these perspectives in the Northwest region of England. While historically, treatment services have been largely geared to harm reduction, a gradual shift is occurring toward a recovery orientation. This shift at the level of the social system may be parallel to the shift that often occurs when an addict is offered compassionate harm reduction approaches in the context of a treatment plan that provides opportunities for participation in a recovery system. Group psychotherapy may be the ideal context in which to offer both opportunities.

McCartney describes in detail some of the interventions that have been implemented in Scotland to support abstinence-based recovery. These interventions include residential treatment, housing, education, and employability services. Although the most sophisticated programs in the United States may also include these kinds of "wraparound" services, we may find comfort in their parallel development in a culture that has previously relied largely on substitution treatments.The second half of this special issue describes specific interventions that have been developed by members of the Recovery Academy. The first article in this section, by Groshkova, Best, and White, provides the kind of research tool that is essential for the systematic study of the impact of groups on recovery from addiction and therefore is a fitting introduction to this section of the issue. Their Recovery Group Participation Scale is applicable to a broad range of recovery groups, including the kinds of groups that are described in the articles that follow.

The article by Logan describes community-based interventions designed to support recovery and rehabilitation of addicts. She reminds us that for opiate addiction in particular, psychosocial interventions have not traditionally been emphasized, and this has been as true in the United Kingdom as in the United States. Logan also reminds us that community interventions are ideally not a "one-size-fits-all" affair.

Yates provides a detailed review of the history of therapeutic communities supporting recovery from addiction and describes how this methodology crossed the Atlantic from the United States to the United Kingdom. An important part of his review details the quintessentially British contributions to the development of therapeutic communities and underscores the use of cross-fertilization of international methods. He concludes his article with suggestions about how therapeutic communities may be instituted in different contexts, such as in the criminal justice system.

The last four articles in this issue offer a delightful variety of group-level interventions that display inspiring creativity. The Calton Athletic Recovery Group (located in Glasgow, Scotland) is an example of a self-supporting group formed around physical and fitness activities and of which the mission is recovery from addiction. This history and development of this activity group is described in the article by Malloch. The group's linkage of physical activity and recovery group activity is an excellent example of the use of combined approaches in supporting recovery from addiction. Sadly the founder of Calton Athletic and the inspiration behind the early recovery movement in Scotland, David Bryce, has passed away since the initial publication of the special issue, but his memory and legacy live on.

The Serenity Café in Edinburgh, Scotland, offers recovering addicts a social space in which to find support for their recovery. How often are the numerous needs of those in recovery assumed to be limited to their treatment (group therapy or otherwise) and/or mutual support groups? Campbell et al. tell the story of how the Serenity Café came into being and how it has emerged as a powerful impetus for community leadership and development in support of recovery from addiction.

A similar story is told by Kidd about service user groups, which are community-based organizations that provide a variety of services to recovering addicts. He describes three such groups in the United Kingdom: UchooseIt, the Basement Project, and Those on the Margins of a Society, or THOMAS. These service user groups share a common mission of providing psychosocial and other support to their constituencies and a flexibility of approach that seeks to meet their users where they are.

As a lovely metaphor for both the process of recovery in the individual addict and the process of moving a culture toward an orientation of recovery, Livingston et al. write about a mountaineering group that evolved in North Wales to serve the needs of recovering addicts. The group, called Drug and Alcohol Recovery Expeditions, or DARE, had to follow its own path of funding, training, and implementation. I suggest that these are issues that all of us can identify with in the evolution of each of our programs.

In this spirit, we hope that the readers of this book, especially those outside of the United States and the United Kingdom, who are working on innovative areas of recovery from addiction, will consider joining the authors of these papers in reporting on their experience, strength and hope. Otherwise, recovery from addiction may be seen as an American invention, with the United Kingdom slowly trying to catch up with nobody else very interested. We trust that this book demonstrates the power and utility of carrying a message of recovery across political boundaries.

Jeffrey D. Roth MD, FAGPA, FASAM
Editor-in-Chief

Recovery and Public Policy: Driving the Strategy by Raising Political Awareness

DAVID BEST

Center for Criminal Justice and Policing, University of the West of Scotland, Hamilton, Lanarkshire, Scotland, United Kingdom

GRACE BALL

Aberdeenshire Alcohol and Drug Partnership, Aberdeen, Scotland, United Kingdom

In both Scotland and England, recovery has emerged as a key concept in public policy and has informed the national strategies in each country. This high-level commitment has provided a major opportunity for the establishment of "recovery-oriented systems of care" in each country but with differences in both the content of the policy and in the mechanisms for implementation. This article discusses questions around implementation and the issue of time scales, with implications for changing cultures and practices in provider agencies and commissioning practices at a local level. Much of this debate concerns attempts to operationalize "recovery" at an individual level and to create meaningful measures of recovery process and outcome. The overview and discussion component will review the challenges faced in attempting to translate recovery policy at a national level into meaningful systems at a local level and the likely impact this will have on individuals and communities attempting to initiate their own recovery journeys.

RATIONALE: WHAT IS THE BENEFIT OF HAVING A NATIONAL DRUG POLICY THAT EMPHASIZES RECOVERY?

White (2008) has called for a transition to a recovery model for treatment characterized by the switch from an acute model of care to a chronic model that recognizes that recovery journeys are a long-term undertaking that involve families and communities and that go beyond the management of acute health issues to broader questions of personal development and growth. This transition also entails fundamental changes in the commissioning and management of services and systems (Lamb, Evans, & White, 2009) and is an ongoing process of culture change, retraining, and refocusing of specialist treatment provision that will take time and involve clear leadership, vision, and direction. That vision has been offered in both Scotland and England by the publication of national drug policies that have emphasized "recovery" as a core pillar of both conceptualizing and addressing addiction problems. This article assesses the impact that both of these policies have had and identifies "translation" issues around implementing a recovery vision at a locality level.

ENGLAND AS A CASE STUDY

In England, there are two core documents, the first published in 2008 and the second in 2010. We will examine these in turn. The UK drug strategy *Drugs: Protecting Families and Communities—2008–2018* (Home Office, 2008) involved both a strategy and an action plan with four key areas of activity that involve protecting communities through tackling supply, crime, and antisocial behavior, preventing harm to children and young people, delivering new approaches to drug treatment and social reintegration, and public information campaigns, communications, and community engagement. The recovery approach has ramifications in two of these areas—around new approaches to treatment and in community engagement, while there is also considerable overlap with the children and young people agenda, particularly for children of drug-using parents. Among the key objectives of the UK drug strategy that are relevant are:

- developing a package of support to help people in drug treatment to complete treatment and to reestablish their lives by ensuring local arrangements are in place to refer people from job centers to sources of housing advice and advocacy and appropriate treatment;
- using opportunities presented by the benefits system to support people in reintegrating into society and gaining employment, with a commitment to

examine further how claimants can be encouraged to engage with treatment and other services; and

- piloting new approaches that allow a more flexible and effective use of resources, including individual budgets to meet treatment and wider support needs.

The implementation of the UK strategy is divided into 3-year phases with an action plan for 2008–2011 currently in operation. Within the treatment component, the objectives set include:

- pilots and guidance around injectable heroin, contingency management, and the use of mutual support networks;
- access to employment programs for drug users in receipt of benefits;
- improved access to housing for drug users in treatment;
- system change pilots assessing (among other things) end-to-end planning and delivery of individual treatment packages; and
- a renewed focus on outcomes.

Specifically for recovery, the UK strategy asserted that:

> The goal of all treatment is for drug users to achieve abstinence from their drug—or drugs—of dependency. In order to deliver against all the treatment system actions in the drug strategy, partnerships will recognize the need to have recovery as the bed rock of all commissioning decisions.

This document has been updated with the *Drug Strategy 2010: Reducing Demand, Restricting Supply, Building Recovery: Supporting People to Live a Drug-Free Life* (Her Majesty's Government, 2010). Not only is recovery elevated to the title of the document, but in the foreword, Home Secretary Teresa May, MP, states: "A fundamental difference between this strategy and those that have gone before is that instead of focusing primarily on reducing the harms caused by drug misuse, our approach will be to go much further and offer every support for people to choose recovery as an achievable way out of dependency" (Her Majesty's Government, 2010, p. 2). From the introduction onward, the language is of a "fundamentally different approach to tackling drugs and an entirely new ambition to reduce drug use and dependence" (Her Majesty's Government, 2010, p. 3).

One of the three core themes of the strategy is "building recovery in communities," with the other main themes around reducing demand and supply. The role of recovery has thus gained momentum and is considerably more overt. The document calls for the generation of recovery champions at a community, therapeutic, and strategic level within a "whole systems approach." There is an increasing recognition of the community as the key locale for recovery activity and the explicit recognition that "recovery can be contagious" (Her Majesty's Government, 2010, p. 21).

In terms of an implementation plan, the 2010 strategy asserts that "we will encourage local areas not to commission services in isolation, but to jointly commission and deliver 'end to end' support. They need to build close links between community, in-patient and residential treatment and rehabilitation providers, who in turn need to forge close links with aftercare services" (Her Majesty's Government, 2010, p. 20). The strategy explicitly endorses "active promotion and support of local mutual aid networks such as Alcoholics and Narcotics Anonymous" (Her Majesty's Government, 2010, p. 21). The responsibility for delivery is devolved to local levels to plan and implement.

The shift is made explicit from the Home Secretary's introduction, the language of the article is suffused with the recovery lexicon, and recovery has succeeded treatment as the key motif for the management of adult drug problems. Although there is not an operational plan for national implementation or for performance management, there is a move to locality ownership as part of the focus on local communities. Equally important is the last quotation emphasizing mutual aid groups and aftercare, and the core role of recovery champions and recovery communities. Further discussion of the implementation of recovery strategies will be undertaken following a brief overview of the Scottish recovery model.

RECOVERY POLICY IN SCOTLAND

In Scotland, the focus was also explicitly around recovery with the publication of *The Road to Recovery: A New Approach to Tackling Scotland's Drug Problem* (Scottish Government, 2008), which produced a number of definitions for recovery, including *"a process through which an individual is enabled to move from their problem drug use, towards a drug-free lifestyle as an active and contributing member of society."* The origins of the recovery agenda in drugs in Scotland were inspired in part by the success of the Scottish Recovery Network for mental health, which had been seen to have played a major role in addressing stigma issues and in working with providers and commissioners to transform local systems to a recovery-oriented model. The commitment to recovery included the assertion that the primary purpose of all services was recovery, although there was no action plan or operationalization of any of the recovery objectives. As with mental health, much of the responsibility for implementation was devolved to a new organization, the Scottish Drugs Recovery Consortium (SDRC), set up under the strategy with the aim of working with the local commissioning systems (alcohol and drug partnerships [ADPs]) to implement recovery approaches and models. The SDRC was provided with £300,000 to become established as an independent charity but one that would work with the Scottish Government in implementing recovery processes and practices.

Following the launch of the strategy, the Scottish Government also commissioned a review of the evidence base around recovery (Best et al., 2010), which included a research framework to specify key areas for development. The aim of this piece of work was to identify the key gaps in knowledge that could potentially be addressed locally.

WHAT DO THE POLICY COMMITMENTS TO RECOVERY IN ENGLAND AND SCOTLAND MEAN, AND WHAT HAS BEEN ACHIEVED?

It is now explicit in both settings that there is a policy that is committed to a recovery philosophy and recognition that this involves fundamental changes in culture, systems, and practice. In both countries, the policy is keen to acknowledge the gains of the treatment models that had previously dominated and to assert the continuity of achievements around harm reduction and acute care models. So what does this mean in practice? Both policy documents are light on implementation planning, with this evolving to a locality level through directors of public health in England and to the SDRC in Scotland. In neither setting is there any attempt to articulate what success would look like or to establish quantifiable targets for numbers initiating or sustaining recovery journeys. Similarly, both policies offer relatively little in the way of practical guidance to commissioners about how to implement or measure recovery.

Why should this be? In England, there is recognition that recovery is an individualized and personal experience that does not readily fall into "diagnostic"-type measures and so the model is more of a direction of travel and offers guidance in the form of a philosophy and model rather than through process targets. The broader change mechanisms of a localized model of oversight and the introduction of outcomes monitoring through "payment by results" has not clarified these questions of what success might look like for individuals, for their families, and for communities. Likewise, similar concerns arise about outcome-based commissioning in terms of the identification of successful recovery-oriented services and larger treatment systems. However, the English strategy is extremely recent and a consultation exercise is underway to consider issues of implementation.

In Scotland, the Road to Recovery strategy is now well established, yet we continue to grapple with many of the same issues around what it is that should be achieved and how it should be measured. The SDRC has been charged with identifying examples of recovery success and attempting to learn lessons from this, but there is no clear commitment to attempting to measure recovery success for individuals or at the level of localities. Our attention will now turn to the question of what the latter might look like—and the question of whether ADPs in Scotland and drug and alcohol action teams (DAATs) in England are good candidates for recovery-oriented systems of care (ROSCs).

LOCALITY IMPLEMENTATION AS RECOVERY-ORIENTED SYSTEMS OF CARE

In 2009, the Center for Substance Abuse Treatment (CSAT) defined an ROSC as "a coordinated network of community-based services and supports that is person-[centered] and builds on the strengths and resilience of individuals, families, and communities to achieve abstinence and improved health, wellness, and quality of life for those with or at risk of alcohol and drug problems" (p. 22). The CSAT article also defines an ROSC as relying on community-based services and supports, as involving collaborative decision making and continuity of services and supports, and as having multiple stakeholder involvement.

The CSAT guidance (2009) reports the perception that "recovery-oriented systems of care are as complex and dynamic as the process of recovery itself" and that "services should optimally be provided in flexible, unbundled packages that evolve over time to meet the changing needs of recovering individuals" (p. 2). However, the report suggests 17 elements of ROSCs. They include that systems are anchored in the communities and provide continuity of care, are based on partnership–consultant relationships, and are culturally responsive and responsive to personal belief systems. Crucially from a systems point of view, there is a commitment to peer-recovery support systems, and CSAT recommends that the system is inclusive of the voices and experiences of recovering individuals and their families within an integrated service provision. From an implementation perspective, it also recommends ongoing monitoring and outreach within a model that is outcomes driven, research based, and adequately and flexibly financed.

When Lamb, Evans, and White (2009) attempted to initiate recovery in Philadelphia, the key stages included an inventory of relationships in the system, the establishment of a recovery advisory committee to develop a recovery definition, a statement of recovery values and a vision document, all stakeholders participating in mapping out a process of transformation, increasing recovery representation within addiction treatment agency decision making, and celebrating the role of recovering families and individuals with recovery events. However, there was recognition that this process of transformation would take time and that it would involve the strategic buy-in and ownership in a process of change. This also involves a more closely aligning commissioning process with broader community development goals to ensure that the model was not too narrowly focused on addiction issues and was not sufficiently integrated into wider community regeneration activities.

CSAT (2009) has reported that where recovery communities become established there must be adequate provision of housing, employment, and social support. Employment and stable housing have also been found to improve self-esteem and to support reintegration into mainstream society. The CSAT document outlines 19 principles for the implementation of ROSCs, including continuity of care, the inclusion of family and partners in the treatment process, the inclusion of the voices and experiences of the person in recovery, and a commitment to peer-based recovery support systems. It is important to note that CSAT has articulated this overview as principles rather than as a definition, and this makes it hard for policymakers to create simple performance measures of recovery that retain the values of being "culturally responsive" and locally driven. In other words, the commitment toward the principles of localism and community determination per se limits the ability for centralized performance management and control.

WHO IS IN RECOVERY?

An additional challenge for the implementation of a recovery strategy is the problem of operationalizing recovery as a personal state to quantify how often it has been achieved. As many individuals will describe recovery as an ongoing process and not as a state, and as one that is personal, it is not obvious that:

- It means the same for different people.
- It means the same for an individual at different points in their recovery journey.
- There are hard indicators that can be ascribed by an external observer.

Where definitions have been produced, this complexity is acknowledged and addressed—in the United States, the Betty Ford Institute Consensus Panel has defined recovery as *"a voluntarily maintained lifestyle characterized by sobriety, personal health and citizenship"* (Betty Ford Institute Consensus Panel, 2007, p. 222). A subsequent panel meeting in the United Kingdom produced an equivalent definition of *"voluntarily sustained control over substance use which [maximizes] health and well-being and participation in the rights, roles and responsibilities of society"* (UK Drug Policy Commission [UKDPC], 2008, p. 6). Yet the concern persists that definitions do little to convey the sense of empowerment and ownership that is intrinsic to the principles of recovery. In other words, the recognition that recovery is lived experience that is personal and will shift over the course of a recovery journey is not consistent with an expert-driven set of criteria, particularly where these include terms such as "sobriety" and "responsibilities." Both of these terms have provoked concerns from a harm reduction perspective among staff in the United Kingdom who have argued that recovery is a political movement about state benefits and unemployment and that it will force people into work when they are not ready and will favor abstinence-oriented interventions.

The report, *Drug Dependence Treatment: Sustained Recovery Management*, by the United Nations Office on Drugs and Crime (2008) provides a strong rationale for a recovery model:

> *Drug-dependent persons frequently experience crises in the areas of medical, psychological, social, vocational, and legal well-being, partly due to their particular vulnerability related to negative health and social consequences of drug use and often co-occurring disorders. In addition, they face the social [stigmatization] and punitive barriers that often hamper sustained recovery and social reintegration ... Therefore, a continuum of care approach, addressing a range of areas, is especially necessary for sustainable rehabilitation and social reintegration efforts.* (p. 22)

White (2007) has described the specialist treatment approach as focusing on an "acute" form of provision that emphasizes symptom management, an approach that is primarily clinical and based on a diagnostic process and an underlying clinical model. In contrast, White (2007) argues that a recovery model assumes that the clinical component is a necessary but not sufficient requirement for addressing the complexity and longevity of addiction, based on the recognition that "stable" recovery will typically take place a number of years after the cessation of the problem behavior and the acute phase of treatment. White and Kurtz (2006) have argued that typically, for opiate users, there is a period of around 5 to 7 years after the last use of heroin before long-term stability of recovery, yet have asserted that rarely are the support systems available consistent with this model, focusing primarily on the acute phase of needs. Furthermore, the recovery approach would emphasize a more holistic model in which experiential and interpersonal components are given equivalent prominence to the remediation or management of physical or psychiatric pathologies.

The advent of recovery policies in England and Scotland has coincided with increased localized activity in this area, but a research body is only slowly emerging, provoking skepticism about its academic heritage and viability and a lack of a consistent evidence base around a "what works" agenda for recovery. The sense in the United Kingdom is that much of the generation of a recovery "movement" has been based on "bottom up" community development and that it has been the pressure from recovery groups and communities that has influenced the development of the recovery-oriented policies. This has significant implications for the provider agencies that are having to adapt their processes and philosophies to something that they often regard as poorly articulated and insufficiently operationalized.

The English and Scottish strategies are both couched in the language of hope—the Scottish strategy stretching ambitions for change into abstinence. Both strategies recognize the importance of children of drug- or alcohol-using parents, with the development of work that examines the impact of childhood stress and future functioning as an adult. However, their commitment to communities and families as the locus of recovery is a challenge to organizational cultures based on a specialist body of knowledge and expertise that has developed over years of expanding drug treatment. For these organizations and for the commissioners who are charged with implementing the strategy at a local level, the huge challenge is how to know what would constitute signs of success and what measures and indicators should be in place. In both Scotland and England, considerable time and resource has been expended on developing treatment monitoring systems to enable central control of numbers in treatment, waiting times, early engagement, and effective retention. There is both a cultural and philosophical dimension to implementation alongside a concern of "not throwing the baby out with the bathwater" concerning the transition to explicitly recovery-focused approaches.

MEASURING RECOVERY IMPLEMENTATION AND ITS IMPACT ON TREATMENT EFFECTIVENESS

The CSAT, in its "Guiding Principles and Elements of Recovery-Oriented Systems of Care" (2009), sets out 12 "guiding principles" of recovery and suggests that "there are many pathways to recovery; recovery is self-directed and empowering; recovery involves a personal recognition of the need for change and transformation; recovery is holistic; recovery has cultural dimensions; recovery exists on a continuum of improved health and wellness; recovery emerges from hope and gratitude; recovery involves a process of healing and self-redefinition; recovery involves addressing discrimination and transcending shame and stigma; recovery is supported by peers and allies; recovery involves (re)joining and (re)building a life in the community; recovery is a reality" (pp. 1–2). The CSAT report goes on to assert that the epidemiological evidence would suggest that "on average, 58% individuals with chronic substance dependence achieve sustained recovery" (CSAT, p. 21).

This provides—as do the definitions proposed by the Betty Ford Institute Consensus Group (2007) and more recently in the United Kingdom by the UKDPC (2008)—some possibility for operationalizing what is meant by recovery, with full recovery involving:

- abstinence from all illicit drug use and alcohol;
- improved quality of life and well-being; and
- engagement in meaningful activities

It is in principle possible that "hard" indicators for at least the first and last of these could be generated based on biomarkers and indicators of employability. Although there are no "objective" measures of quality of life, there are standardized measures such as the brief indicator developed by the World Health Organization (2004). One of the main challenges about this approach is to ensure that there is a switch in assessment and care reviewing from a primarily pathology-based approach to one based on strengths and positive aspirations and expectations (Best & Gilman, 2010), with the resulting impact on worker philosophy and clinical practices.

There remain two problems—the first is about the principles of recovery (how to capture the positive and personal components outlined by the CSAT)—and the second is about who we measure. Although there is some evidence for medication-maintained recovery (White & Mojer-Torres, 2010), many of those in recovery are not in contact with treatment services—and indeed, a proportion will never have had contact with treatment services.

Local areas are considering what recovery means to them at a local level, with resulting implications for process change away from punitive or acute models of care, which focus on symptom management, to what happens to individuals as they move along a recovery journey, how this can be measured, and how a broad recovery philosophy can be reconciled with health and criminal justice targets around engagement and retention. The model proposed below offers a mechanism for initiating this process.

Best and Gilman (2010) have argued that one framework for delivering this would be around the following:

1. The quality of life of people in recovery: the primary measure of recovery functioning to assess life quality among populations engaged in treatment and those involved in recovery communities.
2. Recovery effects on families: assessing the resulting impact on social costs associated with children of substance-using parents.
3. Growth of recovery communities: the number and diversity of recovery groups available in a locality and the level of engagement by people in recovery with those groups.

4. Evidence of the impact of recovery groups: what recovery groups have to do to give something back to their local communities and what impact this has on the overall functioning of that community.
5. Achieving "tipping points" in local communities: where active recovery champions become sufficiently visible and active so that the perceptions and beliefs of local communities begin to change.

To do this will involve creating a new set of metrics and measures that attempt to combine individual-level effects of recovery with family effects and wider social effects. Thus, what is being suggested is to build a UK equivalent of the recovery indicators proposed by White (2008). This will also include assessments of local environmental factors, as recently undertaken in the "Taking the Temperature" work by the Young Foundation (2010) to measure the functioning of local communities. Thus, the measures that will be proposed are:

- individual factors for people in recovery both in treatment and engaged with community recovery groups (quality of life, engagement with criminal justice system, abstinence, engagement in meaningful activities);
- family functioning (number and proportion of children in care or at risk, with parental substance use as the risk factor);
- diversity in type and uptake of community recovery groups and the number and activities of visible recovery champions in the local areas;
- rates of unemployment and disability living allowance attributable to substance misuse; and
- general sense of community satisfaction and well-being and perceptions and stigma and status of substance users.

While we are at an early stage in the evolution of such a collection of outcome measures, these will combine personal and self-reported aspects of recovery with broader family and community-level impact indicators.

CONCLUSION

The policy foundations for recovery are strong in both England and Scotland, with apparent cross-party support for a recovery agenda embedded within a wider agenda around community reintegration and development. In both countries, the extant drug strategies provide a broad set of objectives and goals—in England supplemented by guidance to commissioners—but with the detail largely left to the locality systems of DAATs in England and ADPs in Scotland. This creates a pressing need for meaningful performance indicators that can map the progress of implementation of recovery in local areas.

The evidence from areas that have attempted to implement recovery systems—most famously Philadelphia in the United States (Lamb, Evans, & White, 2009) but more recently in the city of Salford in the United Kingdom (Wisely, 2010)—has yielded three primary questions that need to be answered:

1. How many people are in recovery in and out of treatment services?
2. Does the organizational culture of treatment services support recovery journeys as well as possible?
3. Is the overall treatment system recovery oriented and designed to maximize the stability of recovery?

The Best and Gilman (2010) model above attempts to initiate a UK model for testing at least some of these questions in the wider context of recovery as a core aspect of community regeneration. We have been provided with drug strategies in Scotland and England that offer a huge opportunity for change—it is our challenge to test whether we can translate this into meaningful and consistent delivery across a wide range of services and systems.

REFERENCES

Best, D., & Gilman, M. (2010, February 15). Recovering happiness. *Drink and Drug News*, pp. 7–8.

Best, D., Rome, A., Hanning, K., White, W., Gossop, M., & Taylor, A. (2010). *Research for recovery: A review of the drugs evidence base* (Scottish Government Social Research). Edinburgh, Scotland: Scottish Government.

Betty Ford Institute Consensus Panel. (2007). What is recovery? A working definition from the Betty Ford Institute. *Journal of Substance Abuse Treatment, 33,* 221–228.

Center for Substance Abuse Treatment. (2009). *Guiding principles and elements of recovery-oriented systems of care: What do we know from the research?* U.S. Department of Health and Human Sciences. Retrieved from http://www.samhsa.gov

Her Majesty's Government. (2010). *Drug Strategy 2010: Restricting demand, reducing supply, building recovery.* London, United Kingdom: Home Office.

Home Office. (2008). *Drugs: Protecting families and communities—2008–2018.* London, United Kingdom: Author.

Lamb, R., Evans, A., & White, W. (2009). *The role of partnership in recovery-oriented systems of care: The Philadelphia experience.* Unpublished manuscript.

Scottish Government. (2008). *The road to recovery: A new approach to tackling Scotland's drug problem.* Edinburgh, Scotland: Scottish Government.

UK Drug Policy Commission. (2008). *Recovery consensus statement.* Retrieved from http://www.ukdpc.org.uk/Recovery_Consensus_Statement.shtml

United Nations Office on Drugs and Crime. (2008). *Drug dependence treatment: Sustained recovery management*. Retrieved from http://www.unodc.org/treatnet

White, W. (2007). Addiction recovery: Its definition and conceptual boundaries. *Journal of Substance Abuse Treatment, 33*(3), 229–241.

White, W. (2008). Toward a philosophy of choice: A new era of addiction treatment. *Counselor, 9*(1), 38–43.

White, W., & Kurtz, E. (2006). The varieties of recovery experience. *International Journal of Self-Help and Self-Care, 3*(1/2), 21–61.

White, W., & Mojer-Torres, L. (2010). Recovery-oriented methadone maintenance. Baltimore, MD: Alcohol Technology Transfer Center.

Wisely, C. (2010). Salford: Toward a recovery-oriented city. *Safer Communities, 9*(4), 40–50.

World Health Organization. (2004). The World Health Organization Quality of Life—WHOQOL BREF. Retrieved from http://www.who.int/substance_abuse/research_tools/en/english_whoqol.pdf

Young Foundation. (2010). *Taking the temperature of local communities: The Wellbeing and Resilience Measure (WARM)*. The Young Foundation. Retrieved from www.youngfoundation.org

The Evolution of a UK Evidence Base for Substance Misuse Recovery

TEODORA GROSHKOVA

National Addiction Center, Institute of Psychiatry, King's College London, London, England, United Kingdom

DAVID BEST

Center for Criminal Justice and Policing, University of the West of Scotland, Hamilton, Lanarkshire, Scotland, United Kingdom

This article examines the academic sources and origins of the "recovery movement" in the drugs field in the United Kingdom and considers a series of disparate evidence sources that have been applied and used in this regard. Only two of these originate in traditional addictions materials—treatment outcome and cohort studies—with the remaining studies reviewed coming from a range of other areas. In particular, the sources include a switch in focus from the specialist treatment clinic to the community, and from the therapeutic to the more broadly social. The framework for this approach is explicitly developmental and attends to the published research around crime careers and addiction careers. The final sections of the article review recent UK addiction recovery research and assess where we are and what we currently know—and as a consequence the key gaps and the methodological questions that need to be addressed.

INTRODUCTION AND RATIONALE

There has been considerable discussion about the growth of a "recovery movement" in the addictions field in the United Kingdom, prompted by public policy shifts in Scotland and England and by increasing interest and activity at the community level in self-help, mutual aid, and the emergence of "communities of recovery." The academic rationale for this shift in policy and practice, where one is cited, has been an eclectic mix of evidence primarily related to alcohol (and in particular to Alcoholics Anonymous [AA]), the recovery movement in the mental health field, some recent U.S. evidence around personal recovery and recovery-oriented systems, and more diverse sources including positive psychology, community development, and developmental criminology. This article attempts to contextualize these sources in the context of published and current research that has been undertaken in the United Kingdom and attempts to provide an overview of where this leaves us in terms of a "UK recovery evidence base" and what key issues remain outstanding. The method employed is to review the key studies and models that have been cited in the limited UK recovery research literature relating to alcohol and drug addiction in recent years and to identify issues arising for the generation of a meaningful and coherent research program to develop our understanding in the United Kingdom.

EVIDENCE BASE ORIGINS AND COHORT STUDIES

The research literature on recovery is based on three main data sources: studies of natural recovery, longitudinal cohort studies, and treatment outcome studies. Let us start with the overall picture of the origins of the UK's research base around long-term recovery. To date, only a handful of longitudinal studies addressing the core aspects of the question of "what happens to drug users" have been reported in the research literature. In the alcohol field, one of the first documented longitudinal recovery experiences was the Addiction Research Unit's long-term follow-up project led by Griffith Edwards. In 1968 to 1970, 90 men referred to the Maudsley outpatient clinic for drinking problems were recruited into a controlled trial (Edwards et al., 1977) and then followed up and interviewed at multiple points (Edwards et al., 1986, 1987, 1988). Interview data gathered at the 10-year point evidenced that among a variety of possible outcome patterns, a substantial proportion of individuals had managed to stably move away from dependent drinking, and the authors concluded that 5 years was a key marker of stable alcohol recovery. In a subsequent analysis, Edwards and colleagues (1988) established that none of 25 baseline variables relating to such issues as childhood background, social stability, marital adjustment, personality, or intensity of drinking had much ability to predict either the drinking or other aspects of overall group outcome.

Outside the United Kingdom, longitudinal studies of cohorts with previous addiction treatment contact have focused on the long-range course of addiction and factors that are related to the different aspects and stages in the addiction career. Fifteen years before Edwards et al.'s (1977) study at the

Maudsley, Vaillant (1973) had explored similar terrain with 100 New York City male addicts admitted to Lexington Hospital in 1952 and 1953. The majority of the sample was found to have relapsed after leaving Lexington, but drug use trends over time were toward reduced opiate use. Vaillant (1973) found that 22% were abstinent at the 5-year follow-up point and 37% were abstinent at the 10-year point.

In a naturalistic study of alcohol users, Vaillant (1983) recruited 400 schoolboys who were then followed from age 14 years to 47 years. At some point in time, 110 developed alcohol dependence. Of those, 49 became abstinent for a year or more, and three factors, among others, were identified to have predicted abstinence in this sample: (1) finding a substitute dependency to compete with alcohol use (e.g., meditation); (2) obtaining new social supports (e.g., a grateful employer or a new marriage); and (3) inspirational group membership (e.g., discovering a sustained source of hope, inspiration, and self-esteem in fundamentalist religion or AA). The same factors have emerged in a literature review of remission from misuse of tobacco, food, opiates, and alcohol (Stall & Biernacki, 1986).

NATURAL RECOVERY STUDIES

Natural recovery research has documented cases of individuals who have overcome a range of drug problems without treatment (e.g., Cunningham, 2000; Klingemann, 1991; O'Donnell, Voss, & Clayton, 1976; Robins, 1973; Scharse, 1966; Winick, 1962). The earliest evidence of natural recovery came from Charles Winick's "maturing out" study published in 1962. Winick traced the official records of addicts in files of the Federal Bureau of Narcotics, and data he sourced showed that as addicts approached ages 35 to 40 years, they tended to drop out of the files, which suggested that some transformational life processes had occurred, similar to the ones affecting adolescents maturing out of juvenile delinquency. In 1964 and 1965, Robert Scharse asked known addicts in treatment at East Los Angeles Halfway to identify and locate friends who had used heroin with them but had since given it up. By this method, Scharse identified 71 ex-users and interviewed 40 of them in a dual interview situation (both the addict and the ex-user). He found that at least 9 of the 40 interviewed reported that they had experienced physical dependence from heroin and had recovered without formal help (Scharse).

Robins's (1973) study looked at the patterns of drug use of U.S. soldiers returning from Vietnam. A sample of 898 men who had returned from Vietnam in 1971 was interviewed in 1972 from 8 to 12 months after their return. Approximately 20% of the enlisted men had been dependent on heroin while in Vietnam. Upon return, only 10% of those addicted in Vietnam had reported using drugs between the time of their return and the interview, and only 1% had been readdicted. At the time of the interview, only 2% (8% of those who were dependent users in Vietnam) had reported continued drug use. Veterans have done equally well regardless of whether they have sought addiction treatment upon their return or not. Some further support for these findings is provided by a study by Sobell, Campbell, and Sobell (1996), who reported rates of 75% and 77% recovery without formal help for drinkers in remission. Cunningham (2000) assessed recovery from a range of substances and reported that the use of any formal treatment ranged from 43.1% for cannabis to 90.7% for heroin, with 59.7% of cocaine users seeking formal treatment at some point in their recovery journeys. In other words, many people have achieved recovery through their own volition and with strategies that do not necessitate formal treatment interventions.

Further research has focused on the typology of natural recovery. Klingemann (1991), in a qualitative study of 30 formerly alcohol-dependent users and 30 formerly heroin-dependent users in Switzerland in 1988, identified a typology of motivation to stop characterizing three major stages of the "autoremission" process. At first, in the language of AA, one group of recoverers was described as "hitting bottom" (e.g., experiencing physical, interpersonal, and psychological collapse). Within this group, one subsample was characterized by Klingemann as "cross-road types," who act on the basis of a single crisis (such as health or psychological problems); another subsample consisted of "pressure-sensitive types," who reacted positively to social pressure, which forced them to choose between a life of conformity or an addiction career. In contrast to the "hitting bottom" group, which could usually define a specific turning point, another group was characterized as slowly and harmoniously drifting out of addiction. Their motivation to quit was based on positive changes in their social environment. Yet another group was described as having had esoteric or religious experiences as turning points.

A more recent study of natural recovery from substance dependence and the unfolding social factors was carried out by Granfield and Cloud (2001). This study involved semistructured interviews with 46 formerly drug- or alcohol-dependent persons who have recovered without treatment, including participation in 12-step groups, for their substance dependencies. Many of the participants in their study felt that the "ideological" base of some self-help programs was inconsistent with their own philosophies of life. The subjects in the study by Granfield and Cloud (2001) also felt that some self-help groups encouraged dependence and that associating with other alcoholics would probably make recovery more difficult. In summarizing their findings, Granfield and Cloud (2001) reported that the respondents in their study discounted the use of self-help groups because they saw themselves as "efficacious people who often prided themselves on their past accomplishments. Granfield and Cloud (2001) added to the social context notion of recovery by noting that many of the respondents in their sample had a great deal to lose if they continued their substance abuse. They noted that the subjects in their study "had jobs, supportive families, high school and college credentials, and other social supports that gave them reasons to alter their drug-taking behavior," and they added that "having much to lose" gave their respondents "incentives to transform their lives" (p. 1555).

TREATMENT OUTCOME STUDIES

What has so far been presented is "outcome" of natural recovery. This picture must be supplemented by information about what happens to the treatment and recovery populations. The evidence for positive outcome for intensive, abstinence-based interventions is reasonably encouraging. The Drug Abuse Reporting Program found that 53% of patients who had been daily users of opioids before treatment were not daily opioid users at 1 year, and continued improvement was observed over time until Year 6 when the proportion of nonusers stabilized at 58% for "any" use and at 75% for "daily" use. At the time of the 12-year follow-up, the favorable outcome was retained, with the proportion of nonusers slightly increasing to 61% and 76% for "any" use and for "daily" use, respectively (Simpson & Sells, 1990).

During 1995, the English National Treatment Outcome Research Study (NTORS) recruited 1,075 patients from 54 treatment programs (Table 1). One year after intake to treatment, outcome data were obtained for 769 patients (72%). Subsequent follow-ups at 2 years and 4 to 5 years were conducted with a random stratified sample of patients. At 1-year follow-up, within the residential settings, the percentage of clients from the rehabilitation programs who were abstinent from illicit opiates increased from 27% at intake to 58% at 1-year follow-up, while the proportion of regular users fell from 63% to 33% (Gossop, Marsden, & Stewart, 1998). Gossop, Stewart, Treacy,

TABLE 1 UK Addiction Treatment Outcome Data

	NTORS		DTORS		DORIS
Year of recruitment	March–July 1995		Feb 2006–March 2007		2001
Numbers recruited	1,075 IP, $n = 122$ (11%); RR, $n = 286$ (27%); MR, $n = 209$ (19%); & MMT, $n = 458$ (43%)		1,796		1,007
Settings	54 TPs		342 TPs		33 TPs
Follow-up period	1 Y	2; 4–5 Y	3–5 M	11–13 M	8; 16; 33 M
Follow-up rate	72%	RSS	63%	28%	77% (33 M)
% self-reporting illicit opiates abstinence	56%	49%	44%	49%	15% (33 M)
% employed			11%	16%	20% (33 M)

Y = year; M = month; IP = inpatient; MMT = methadone maintenance treatment; RR = residential rehabilitation; MR = methadone reduction; TP = treatment program; RSS = Random stratified sample.

and Marsden (2002), reporting on the 2-year outcomes from the NTORS, found that 48% of admissions to residential treatment were abstinent from all opiates, with the majority of this group sustaining abstinence during the full 4- to 5-year follow-up period and demonstrating high rates of continuity of abstinence.

The follow-up to NTORS in England—the Drug Treatment Outcomes Research Study (DTORS)—used a 12-month window to assess treatment outcomes, supplemented by a qualitative assessment of "treatment-related issues" and a cost-effectiveness analysis. In total, 1,796 drug users were recruited from 342 agencies across England. Of the initial cohort, 1,131 were successfully followed up at 3 to 5 months, and 504 were followed up at 11 to 13 months. From the Key Implications summary (Home Office Research Report 24, 2009), the conclusion was that DTORS outcomes were equivalent or more positive for treatment effectiveness than those found in NTORS. Employment rates increased from 9% at baseline to 11% at Follow-Up 1 and 16% at Follow-Up 2. However, the proportion of participants classed as unable to work also increased during the course of the study follow-ups. Similarly, offending reduced from a self-reported level of 40% at baseline to 21% at first follow-up and 16% at second follow-up. Among heroin users involved in the baseline interviews, 44% had stopped using at first follow-up and 49% had stopped using at second follow-up, and there were consistent reductions in all of the other major substances assessed during the course of the follow-up periods.

The Scottish Drug Treatment Outcome Research Study (DORIS) was a prospective cohort study that recruited 1,007 drug misusers from 33 agencies, including five prisons, across Scotland. The study involved follow-up assessments at 8 months, 16 months, and 33 months postintake to the study and achieved a 70% follow-up rate at the 33-month follow-up point. Although there were initial improvements to 8 months, these tapered off at the subsequent follow-up points. The authors concluded that, compared with other community programs, residential rehabilitation clients were twice as likely to be abstinent at 33 months, while methadone maintenance treatment was associated with reductions in heroin use but was not successful in promoting abstinence. In an article drawn from the study, McKeganey, Bloor, Robertson, Neale, and McDougall (2006) reported on 695 follow-ups at 33 months and found that only 5.9% of females and 9.0% of males were abstinent in the 90 days prior to interview.

In an analysis of uptake of employment during the period of the DORIS study, McIntosh, Bloor, and Robertson (2008) reported that 20.1% of the follow-up sample (140/695) had been in paid employment since the previous interview. The main predictors of achieving employment were being younger, having lower levels of crime involvement, and receiving support from the treatment agency through training and education or through obtaining a job. Treatment modality was not linked to employment status.

The overall DORIS study report found evidence of a strong association between substance use and crime, and consistent with other studies, reported decreases in acquisitive crime in the treatment population but concluded that these reductions were the consequence of changes in substance use rather than a direct treatment effect on offending behavior.

UK's studies of treatment effectiveness and outcome of substance misuse cover relatively short periods of time (up to 33 months), although the NTORS team followed up a subsample of the original cohort 5 years after admission to treatment. The question arises as to whether relatively short-term studies can inform about the complex processes of stability and change that occur during the life course. Technically, of course, the answer is no. Because both complex temporal processes and the effects of social factors are so prominent, however, these studies demonstrate much of the logic of life course research, which is in focus in the next section, despite their shorter-than-desirable time frames.

STUDIES MEASURING RECOVERY PROCESS

A useful parallel can be seen in research on cocaine use. Waldorf, Reinarman, and Murphy (1991), based on 267 in-depth interviews with heavy cocaine users, found that many addicted people with supportive elements in their lives (a job, family, and other close emotional supports) were able to "walk away" from their very heavy use of cocaine. The authors suggested that the "social context" of drug users' lives might positively influence their ability to discontinue drug use.

In the United Kingdom (Glasgow), McIntosh and McKeganey (2001) interviewed 70 recovering heroin-dependent individuals to gain insight into their views about the recovery process. For the majority of individuals in their sample, the process of overcoming dependent drug use involved multiple attempts to stop. A range of reasons was given for attempting to stop using. What appeared to distinguish individuals, as far as successful and unsuccessful attempts were concerned, was the individual's sense of identity, or what was described as the person's desire and determination to restore a "spoiled identity."

Furthermore, Shewan and Dalgarno (2005), in a longitudinal study of 126 nontreatment heroin users in Glasgow between 1996 and 2000, stressed the importance of the broader social environment while exploring patterns and trends of controlling as a component of "unobtrusive" heroin use. The participants they described in the study were typically experienced users of heroin, among a range of other drugs. Virtually, the complete sample ($n = 124$, 98%) were heroin users, who have been taking the drug for 9 years. In contrast to typical samples of heroin users, levels of educational achievement and work status were high—64% had progressed to levels of education beyond secondary school and 74% were employed—and comparable to those found in the general UK population. Although problems with health and social factors such as family and employment were reported, ongoing problems were rare in this sample, and heroin was not found to be a significant predictor of either context. Furthermore, Davies (1992) has contributed to the argument about the formative power of interactions, stigma, and labels for identity development and change of problematic identities.

DEVELOPMENTAL MODELS OF CHANGE

A lot of major issues in the study of drug and alcohol dependence involve conceptualizing and modeling change. Estimating the effects of a range of biographical factors and other topics requires conceptualization of processes and analysis of longitudinal data. Such a model of change that traces the temporal pathways in the dynamic interplay between life events and problem behaviors is consistent with the "life-course perspective model" of substance use and the related concept of the "turning point," discussed by Hser, Longshore, and Anglin (2007). Key assumptions of this model are that lives unfold over time in long-term pathways or trajectories; that the present cannot be understood without knowledge of the past, including the distant past; and that in addition to the content of trajectories (e.g., family histories, occupational careers), their temporal characteristics also are important (Settersten, 2006). Potentially important temporal characteristics include length of exposure (i.e., the extent to which time in a given state affects outcomes of interest), sequencing (i.e., the extent to which the order in which events or exposures occur affects outcomes of interest), and duration dependence (i.e., the extent to which time in a given state alters the probability of movement to another state).

Hser, Hoffman, Grella, and Anglin (2001) and Hser and colleagues (2007) used longitudinal data to examine predictors of desistance in heroin users followed up during a 33-year window and found that self-efficacy and psychological well-being were predictors of stable recovery. The authors emphasized key developmental concepts such as trajectories and turning points, although they conceded that there was a dearth of information about cessation factors. One of their observations was that career pathways appeared to differ for different substances, with cocaine use increasing through the 20s to early 30s and then declining, but heroin use continuing to increase. In terms of the typology of heroin users developed by Hser and colleagues (2007), the authors differentiated between stable high-level users, decelerating users, and early quitters. The last group (who constituted just under half of their longitudinal sample) had heroin careers of typically less than 10 years. This early quitting population of heroin users had higher frequencies of use in the first 2 to 3 years but then showed marked reductions and abstinence by Year 11.

From the literature on both mental health and crime, a number of studies have explored the potential of taking a "life course" perspective as the key methodological approach. In a series of research articles (e.g., Laub, Nagin, & Sampson, 1998; Sampson & Laub, 1990) and a book (Laub & Sampson, 2003) based on a sample of delinquent males born in the 1920s who were studied intermittently until age 70 years, Sampson and Laub demonstrate that the accumulation of social resources, especially stable jobs and supportive marriages, inhibit adult crime, psychiatric symptoms, and substance misuse/dependence. Long and Vaillant (1984) studied a sample of inner-city men from the time they were children until they were 47 years old. During childhood, boys from unstable homes exhibited substantially higher rates of delinquent behavior and psychiatric symptoms than boys in stable homes. By age 47, however, psychiatric and substance use symptoms were unrelated to childhood family stability. Both studies were based on high-risk samples where elevated rates of psychiatric problems and offending during adulthood would be expected as a result of socioeconomic deprivations and high rates of delinquency. In both samples, however, surprisingly high proportions of study participants were able to overcome their early adversities and be productive and healthy adults. Thus, multiple trajectories describe both samples, with some pathways associated with continued psychiatric vulnerability during adulthood and other pathways demonstrating impressive resilience, and there is little evidence that early risk factors have long-term developmental predictiveness.

For Laub and Sampson (2003), the key predictors of long-term change and growth were structural life events (having a stable relationship and a job), changes in psychological resources (interpersonal skills, life and coping skills, and a change in personal identity), and ageing. In follow-up research, the "good marriage effect" on desistance from crime has been found to be particularly robust and maintains its influence for both men and women (Giordano, Cernkovich, & Rudolph, 2002) in studies using official and self-report data (Blockland & Nieuwbeerta, 2005; Massoglia & Uggen, 2007) and across historical contexts (Bersani, Laub, & Nieuwbeerta, 2009).

The notion of long-term change is not new to the addictions field. More than 50% or more of the daily users of alcohol and other drugs stop using because they "mature out" or as a result of treatment (see White, 2008, for review). There is, however, no cutoff beyond which clients are "safe" from relapse risk. In 2007, Dennis, Foss, and Scott reported on 8-year outcomes among a cohort of 1,326 substance users accessing treatment services; at the 8-year follow-up point, 501 were abstinent from alcohol and illicit drugs (37.8%), of whom only 77 (15.4%) had been abstinent for 5 years or more. A total of 142 individuals (10.7% of the total sample) had been abstinent for at least 3 years. Increasing duration of abstinence was associated with more days in employment, fewer debts, and fewer days of incarceration. The point of recovery stability/durability (point at which the risk for future lifetime relapse drops below 15%) is typically 4 to 5 years of sustained recovery for alcohol dependence but potentially longer for other drug dependencies (e.g., opioid addiction; see White & Kurtz, 2006, for review). Little is known about the dynamics of relapse following a prolonged period of stable recovery (White & Schulstad, 2009).

RECOVERY CAPITAL AND THE MECHANISMS OF LONG-TERM CHANGE

Recovery careers—their initiation and durability—are profoundly influenced by the interaction of problem severity/complexity and "recovery capital." Recovery capital is the quantity and quality of internal and external resources that can be mobilized to initiate and sustain the resolution of severe alcohol and other drug problems (Granfield & Cloud, 1999). Internal assets can be thought of as personal recovery capital, and external assets can be thought of in terms of family and community recovery capital (White & Cloud, 2008).

Recovery capital has its origins in the notion of social capital (Bourdieu, 1998), which meshes with the idea about linked lives and with one of the core principles of life-course perspectives contending that virtually all outcomes of interest are affected by the social networks within which individuals are embedded. One dimension of the effects of social relationships on recovery and relapse is the nature of the recovery individual's network. The risk for relapse following recovery initiation rises in relationship to the density of heavy drug users in one's posttreatment social network and declines in tandem with social network support for abstinence (Best, Ghufran, et al., 2008; Bond, Kaskutas, & Weisner, 2003; Dennis et al., 2007; Mohr, Averna, Kenny, & Del Boca, 2001; Weisner, Matzger, & Kaskutas, 2003).

Individuals recovering from alcohol and drug problems typically use social support through their involvement in self- or mutual-help programs such as those found in 12-step fellowships (Humphreys, 2004; Humphreys, Mankowski, Moos, & Finney, 1999). Involvement in 12-step fellowships (e.g., AA, Narcotics Anonymous) has been related to improvements in remission rates among individuals with substance misuse disorders (Humphreys, 2004; Ritsher, McKellar, Otilingam, & Moos, 2002). Research data from an 8-year outcome study (Moos & Moos, 2004) suggested that continued involvement in self-help programs might produce additional desirable health outcomes. More participation in self-help settings might result in an increased amount of social support experienced by individuals in recovery (Humphreys et al., 1999), and this support has been associated with better outcomes for both abstinence (Noone, Dua, & Markham, 1999) and psychological functioning

(Laudet, Magura, Vogel, & Knight, 2000). However, the lack of stable living environments for some substance-dependent individuals poses significant obstacles to community reintegration, and these obstacles have been over-come by the use of therapeutic communities. Therapeutic communities are homelike environments that differ from traditional treatment settings in that they are residential settings that rely less on professional direction and more on client participation (De Leon, 2000). These environments nurture self-help behavior as individuals live together, participate in work responsibilities, and embrace a collective and supportive lifestyle (Condelli & Hubbard, 1994; De Leon, 1995).

The evidence for effectiveness of peer-based interventions derives in part from a series of studies that looks at recovery management check-up approaches. Scott and Dennis (2009) operationalized recovery manage-ment check-ups as quarterly check-ups that are supplemented by motiva-tional interviewing and treatment linkage and that provide ongoing support. Compared with control clients, participants receiving recovery management check-ups reported more days of abstinence and fewer symptoms of de-pendence or drug-induced problems and were more effectively engaged in treatment. The authors concluded that *"ongoing monitoring, feedback and early re-intervention can be effective methods managing recovery over time"* (Scott & Dennis, 2009, p. 969). This model also provides considerable opti-mism about the possibility of peer-driven recovery management check-ups in which those in recovery deliver the intervention and monitor and support peers earlier in the recovery process.

Another clinical trial method was used by Litt and colleagues (2007) who assessed the benefits of randomizing people to "network support." They found that of 186 participants randomly assigned to network support (NS), case management (CM), or network support plus contingency management (NS + CM), participants in both NS conditions had better outcomes than CM alone. The authors found that *"[t]he addition of just one abstinent person to a social network increased the probability of abstinence for the next year by 27%"* (Litt, Kadden, Kabela-Cormier, & Petry, 2007, p. 550).

RECENT UK RECOVERY RESEARCH

Best and colleagues, in various publications, have pioneered the emerging UK evidence base on recovery in addictions. Their first report (Best, Ghufran, et al., 2008) was based on 107 former heroin users who were recruited op-portunistically from three sources; this report drew heavily from former users working in the addictions field. On average, the group had heroin careers lasting for just under 10 years, punctuated by an average of 2.6 treatment episodes and 3.1 periods of abstinence. When asked what enabled them to finally give up using heroin, the answer was most commonly about "having had enough"—a gradual process of not wanting to live that life any more but also involving an event that was family or health related in many cases and that finally gave them the impetus to make the initial change. However, the key finding from this study was that participants readily differentiated between the factors that allowed them to achieve abstinence and the factors that allowed them to sustain it. The most important factors in sustaining recovery were social network factors (moving away from drug-using friends and support from nonusing friends) and practical factors (accommodation and employment), as well as religious or spiritual factors.

Follow-ups to this initial research examined the pathways to drug and alcohol recovery and the resulting level of psychosocial functioning. Based on three groups (98 primary drinkers, 104 primary heroin users, and 67 individuals reporting problems with both alcohol and drugs), the research group reported on the differences in trajectories of recovery careers among problem substance users and the reasons for achieving and maintaining desistance (Best & Laudet, 2010). Former heroin users reported more rapid escalation to problematic use but much shorter *careers involving daily use than was the case in the alcohol cohort*. Alcohol and heroin users also differed in their self-reported reasons for stopping use, with drinkers more likely to report work and social reasons and drug users to report criminal justice factors. In sustaining abstinence, alcohol users more often reported partner support and drug users peer support and were also more likely to emphasize the need to move away from substance-using friends than was the case for former drinkers. Users of both alcohol and heroin were least likely to cite partner factors in sustaining recovery but were more likely to need to move away from using friends and then to cite reasonable accommodation as crucial in sustaining abstinence.

There are two implications from this study. The first is that it is further evidence of what little knowledge we have of recovery pathways and how they may vary. The evidence from this research is that different substance profiles may have different implications for recovery pathways and routes—and also for the likelihood that people will use either mutual aid groups or formal treatment services. It says, however, little about what the effect of location, gender, ethnicity, age, and other factors might have on recovery pathways. It also says little about nonabstinent recovery.

Extended analysis (Best, Groshkova, et al., in press) looked at the quality of life and recovery in these cohorts. This Birmingham-based group consisted of 132 individuals in medication-maintained recovery and 87 in abstinent recovery, although almost the entire group had received a substitute prescription at some point. Nonmedicated recovery was associated with better quality of life in terms of physical well-being and satisfaction with the lived environment, with fewer physical health symptoms, and with less anxiety about using heroin. However, perhaps the crucial difference was around the social networks of the two groups—the nonmedicated group reported much less contact with current drug users and significantly less time spent with them each week. The overall models of quality of life in both groups suggested that being older was associated with greater quality of life (rather than time since last use) supporting a "maturing out" hypothesis.

In a similar regression-based model based on the Glasgow data, Best, Gow, et al. (in press) assessed recovery and quality of life outcomes. Longer time since last use of alcohol or heroin was associated with significantly better quality of life at the time of interview. One of the key findings reported was the prominent role played by ongoing engagement in meaningful activities. Not only was this associated with better day-to-day functioning (e.g., less anxiety and depression, fewer physical health symptoms, and greater self-esteem and self-efficacy), it was also the single most powerful predictor of overall quality of life in the study. The data did not permit causal inferences, but it appeared that those who were engaged in daily activities—working, training, volunteering, and looking after household—were happier and functioned better than those not engaged in such activates. The second most powerful predictor of quality of life was the number of people in recovery social networks—in other words, being active and having a support network of people in recovery were very powerful predictors of life quality among those in recovery.

IMPLICATIONS AND LIMITATIONS IN OUR CURRENT KNOWLEDGE BASE

This is not a systematic review of the literature on recovery but rather an overview of some of the key research studies and models that have shaped thinking about recovery in the United Kingdom. The purpose of the review is to recognize that treatment outcome studies—and even cohort studies—have played a relatively limited role in conceptualizing recovery, with at least as much emphasis on studies of "natural recovery" or "autoremission" that have used very different methodologies, including recruitment via advertising in local newspapers and population-level sampling. The second key conclusion is that much of the literature that has gained prominence does not have its origins in the addictions field but rather with key areas including criminology, mental health, and the history of community development, in particular through the involvement of mutual aid.

It is this diversity of sources that has also led to a broadening of theoretical constructs of "addiction" and "recovery" to incorporate both developmental and social approaches. This has been a critical development in locating recovery as something that happens largely outside of treatment services. The conclusions drawn by White and Kurtz (2006) that the time to stable recovery is around 5 years after last drug ingestion are consistent with the belief that recovery is something that is a process and one that takes place primarily in the community. White's (2008) argument that a recovery model involves switching from an acute model of care to a chronic or longitudinal one forces a model of recovery that focuses on stabilizing factors such as social networks (Litt, Kadden, Kabela-Cormier, & Petrie, 2009), employment and training, and supportive relationships (Best et al., 2008). While this does not mean that the effectiveness of specialist treatment is diminished in relevance, it would suggest that it is not sufficient to enable an enduring recovery journey, as so necessitates a switch in academic focus to community support and development issues.

What such a shift in perspective necessitates is a refocusing of research attention that is cast in the language and conceptual models of recovery thinking. The work that has been initiated in the United Kingdom has largely been opportunistic in that it has used the retrospective accounts of opportunistic samples of individuals and groups in recovery to reconstruct recovery processes and pathways. The greatest challenges for research are the demands of a "life-course perspective model" that examines the life histories of drug-dependent individuals and studies examining the outcome of events such as addiction treatment. This model raises questions around mechanisms of change—that within a life-course model, there are "windows of opportunity for change" that represent the turning points in a developmental trajectory. The challenge for science is to identify when and why these occur and what makes the changes sustainable. The latter question provokes key questions about the operationalization of the concept of "recovery capital" and what is needed to enable growth in the key areas of personal, social, and community recovery capital (Best & Laudet, 2010). Finally, the core area arising from studies such as that by Litt and colleagues (2007) would suggest the core role of social networks and the impact of sober recovery networks, and a key area for developing the UK evidence base will be around assessing transitions in and impact of recovery networks.

If recovery is about resolving problems in living and rectifying the interactions between the individual and other people, including the larger culture, one of the primary missions as a field is to help emerging recovery communities and document their contribution to individual development, community betterment, and positive social change. Many community settings embody many of our core values, priorities, and goals. Thus, increasing the number and impact of recovery supports in the community is applicable as a guiding ideal. Much work remains to be done to test and expand many of the concepts, characteristics, pathways, and processes described. These include the idea of recovery-oriented systems of care—the transformation of locality services and models to maximize and individualize recovery processes and journeys.

The review of the key studies and the implications for future directions are limited to the extent that they reflect the views of the authors.

This in part reflects the limited interest among UK addiction researchers in the ideas around recovery and in part the early stage of the development of this approach and model. The limitations extend to the selection of materials to be included, which were not derived from a systematic review and which vary markedly in their original aims and methods. This raises further questions about the research methodology that should be preferred and prioritized in recovery research. The dominance of Randomized Control Trial (RCT)-type designs is less appropriate for recovery studies where issues of sampling and research design are more likely to be influenced by issues of access and visibility of recovery groups.

The overall conclusion from this article is that there is a rich diversity of important empirical sources for a recovery model for addiction theory and addiction research in the United Kingdom, and that may provide the basis for a research agenda and philosophy in the United Kingdom.

REFERENCES

Bersani, B., Laub, J., & Nieuwbeerta, P. (2009). Marriage and desistance from crime in the Netherlands: Do gender and socio-historical context matter? *Journal of Quantitative Criminology, 25*, 3–24.

Best, D., Ghufran, S., Day, E., Ray, R., & Loaring, J. (2008). Breaking the habit: A retrospective analysis of desistance factors among formerly problematic heroin users. *Drug and Alcohol Review, 27*(6), 619–624.

Best, D., Gow, J., Knox, T., Taylor, A., Groshkova, T., & White, W. (in press). Mapping the recovery stories of drinkers and drug users in Glasgow: Quality of life and its predictors. *Drug and Alcohol Review*. Manuscript submitted for publication.

Best, D., Groshkova, T., Sadler, J., Day, E., & White, W. (in press). The recovery experiences of a service user group and their peer networks in Birmingham, England. *Alcohol Treatment Quarterly*. Manuscript submitted for publication.

Best, D., & Laudet, A. (2010). *The potential of recovery capital, RSA Projects*. Retrieved from http://www.thersa.org/projects/our-projects/reports/the-potential-of-recovery-capital

Blockland, A., & Nieuwbeerta, P. (2005). The effects of life circumstances on longitudinal trajectories of offending. *Criminology, 43*, 1203–1240.

Bond, J., Kaskutas, L. A., & Weisner, C. (2003). The persistent influence of social networks and Alcoholics Anonymous on abstinence. *Journal of Studies on Alcohol, 64*(4), 579–588.

Bourdieu, P. (1998, December). Utopia of endless exploitation—The essence of neoliberalism. *Le Monde Diplomatique*. Retrieved from http://mondediplo.com/1998/12/08bourdieu

Condelli, W., & Hubbard, R. (1994). Relationship between time spent in treatment and client outcomes from therapeutic communities. *Journal of Substance Abuse Treatment, 11*, 25–33.

Cunningham, J. (2000). Remissions from drug dependence: Is treatment a prerequisite? *Drug and Alcohol Dependence, 59*(3), 211–213.

Davies, J. B. (1992). *The myth of addiction*. London, United Kingdom: Harwood Academic.

De Leon, G. (1995). Therapeutic communities for addictions: A theoretical framework. *International Journal of the Addictions, 30*(12), 1603–1645.

De Leon, G. (2000). *The therapeutic community: Theory, model, and method*. New York, NY: Springer.

Dennis, M. L., Foss, M. A., & Scott, C. K. (2007). An 8-year perspective on the relationship between the duration of abstinence and other aspects of recovery. *Evaluation Review, 31*(6), 585–612.

Edwards, G., Brown, D., Duckitt, A., Oppenheimer, E., Sheehan, M., & Taylor, C. (1986). Normal drinking in a recovered alcohol addict. *British Journal of Addiction, 81*, 127–138.

Edwards, G., Brown, D., Duckitt, A., Oppenheimer, E., Sheehan, M., & Taylor, C. (1987). Outcome of alcoholism: The structure of patient attributions as to what causes change. *British Journal of Addiction, 82*, 533–545.

Edwards, G., Brown, D., Oppenheimer, E., Sheehan, M., Taylor, C., & Duckitt, A. (1988). Long-term outcome for patients with drinking problems: The search for predictors. *British Journal of Addiction, 83*, 917–927.

Edwards, G., Orford, J., Egert, S., Guthrie, S., Hawker, A., Hensman, C., . . . Taylor, C. (1977). Alcoholism: A controlled trial of 'treatment' and 'advice.' *Journal of Studies on Alcohol, 38*, 1004–1031.

Giordano, P., Cernkovich, S., & Rudolph, J. (2002). Gender, crime, and desistance: Toward a theory of cognitive transformation. *American Journal of Sociology, 107*, 990–1064.

Gossop, M., Marsden, J., & Stewart, D. (1998). NTORS at 1 year: The National Treatment Outcome Research Study—Changes in substance use, health, and criminal behaviors 1 year after intake. Retrieved from http://www.dh.gov.uk/prod_consum_dh/groups/dh_digitalassets/@dh/@en/documents/digitalasset/dh_4076746.pdf

Gossop, M., Stewart, D., Treacy S., & Marsden, J. (2002). A prospective study of mortality among drug misusers during a 4-year period after seeking treatment. *Addiction, 97*, 39–47.

Granfield, R., & Cloud, W. (1999). *Coming clean: Overcoming addiction without treatment*. New York, NY: New York University Press.

Granfield, R., & Cloud, W. (2001). Social context and 'natural recovery': The role of social capital in the resolution of drug-associated problems. *Substance Use and Misuse, 36*, 1543–1570.

Home Office Research Report 24. (2009). *The Drug Treatment Outcomes Research Study (DTORS): Final outcomes report* (3rd ed.). Retrieved from http://rds.homeoffice.gov.uk/rds/pdfs09/horr24c.pdf

Hser, Y., Hoffman, V., Grella, C., & Anglin, M. D. (2001). A 33-year follow-up of narcotics addicts. *Archives of General Psychiatry, 58*(5), 503–508.

Hser, Y., Longshore, D., & Anglin, M. D. (2007). The life course perspective on drug use: A conceptual framework for understanding drug use trajectories. *Evaluation Review, 31*(6), 515–547.

Humphreys, K. (2004). *Circles of recovery: Self-help organizations for addictions* (International Research Monographs on Addiction). Cambridge, United Kingdom: Cambridge University Press.

Humphreys, K., Mankowski, E., Moos, R. H., & Finney, J. W. (1999). Do enhanced friendship networks and active coping mediate the effect of self-help groups on substance use? *Annals of Behavioral Medicine, 21,* 54–60.

Klingemann, H. (1991). The motivation for change from problem alcohol and heroin use. *British Journal of Addiction, 86,* 727–744.

Laub, J. H., Nagin, D. S., & Sampson, R. J. (1998). Trajectories of change in criminal offending: Good marriages and the desistance process. *American Sociological Review, 63,* 225–238.

Laub, J. H., & Sampson, R. J. (2003). *Shared beginnings, divergent lives: Delinquent boys to age 70.* Cambridge, MA: Harvard University Press.

Laudet, A. B., Magura, S., Vogel, H., & Knight, E. (2000). Addictions services: Support, mutual aid, and recovery from dual diagnosis. *Community Mental Health Journal, 36*(5), 457–476.

Litt, M. D., Kadden, R. M., Kabela-Cormier, E., & Petry, N. (2007). Changing network support for drinking: Initial findings from the Network Support Project. *Journal of Consulting and Clinical Psychology, 754,* 542–555.

Litt, M. D., Kadden, R. M., Kabela-Cormier, E., & Petry, N. (2009). Changing network support for drinking: Network support project 2-year follow up. *Journal of Consulting and Clinical Psychology, 77*(2), 229–242.

Long, J. V. F., & Vaillant, G. E. (1984). Natural history of male psychological health: XI. Escape from the underclass. *American Journal of Psychiatry, 141,* 341–346.

Massoglia, M., & Uggen, C. (2007). Subjective desistance and the transition to adulthood. *Journal of Contemporary Criminal Justice, 23,* 90–103.

McIntosh, J., Bloor, M. J., & Robertson, M. (2008). The health benefits of reductions in individuals' use of illegal drugs. *Journal of Substance Use, 13*(4), 247–254.

McIntosh, J., & McKeganey, N. (2001). Identity and recovery from dependent drug use: The addict's perspective. *Drugs: Education, Prevention, and Policy, 8,* 47–59.

McKeganey, N. P., Bloor, M. J., Robertson, M., Neale, J., & McDougall, J. (2006). Abstinence and drug abuse treatment: Results from the Drug Outcome Research in Scotland Study. *Drugs: Education, Prevention, and Policy, 13*(6), 537–550.

Mohr, C. D., Averna, S., Kenny, D. A., & Del Boca, F. K. (2001). Getting by (or getting high) with a little help from my friends: An examination of adult alcoholics' friendships. *Journal of Studies on Alcohol, 62*(5), 637–645.

Moos, R., & Moos, B. (2004). Long-term influence of duration and frequency of participation in Alcoholics Anonymous on individuals with alcohol use disorders. *Journal of Consulting and Clinical Psychology, 72,* 81–90.

Noone, M., Dua, J., & Markham, R. (1999). Stress, cognitive factors, and coping resources as predictors of relapse in alcoholics. *Addictive Behaviors, 24,* 687–693.

O'Donnell, J., Voss, H., & Clayton, R. (1976). *Young men and drugs: A nationwide survey.* Washington, DC: National Institute on Drug Abuse.

Ritsher, J. B., McKellar, J. W., Otilingam, P. G., & Moos, R. H. (2002). Psychiatric comorbidity, continuing care, and self-help as predictors of substance abuse remission 5 years after intensive treatment. *Journal of Studies on Alcohol, 63,* 709–715.

Robins, L. N. (1973). *The Vietnam drug user returns*. Washington, DC: U.S. Government Printing Office.

Sampson, R. J., & Laub, J. H. (1990). Crime and deviance over the life course: The salience of adult social bonds. *American Sociological Review*, *55*, 609–627.

Scharse, R. (1966). Cessation patterns among neophyte heroin users. *International Journal of Addictions*, *1*(2), 23–32.

Scott, C. K., & Dennis, M. L. (2009). Results from two randomized clinical trials evaluating the impact of quarterly recovery management checkups with adult chronic substance users. *Addiction*, *104*, 959–971.

Settersten, R. A. (2006). Aging and the life course. In R. H. Binstock & L. K. George (Eds.), *Handbook of aging and the social sciences* (6th ed., pp. 3–19). San Diego, CA: Academic.

Shewan, D., & Dalgarno, P. (2005). Evidence for controlled heroin use? Low levels of negative health and social outcomes among nontreatment heroin users in Glasgow (Scotland). *British Journal of Health Psychology*, *10*, 33–48.

Simpson, D. D., & Sells, S. B. (Eds.). (1990). *Opioid addiction and treatment: A 12-year follow-up*. Malabar, FL: Robert E. Krieger.

Sobell, L., Campbell, J. A., & Sobell, M. B. (1996). Recovery from alcohol problems with and without treatment: Prevalence in two population surveys. *American Journal of Public Health*, *7*, 966–972.

Stall, R., & Biernacki, P. (1986). Spontaneous remission from the problematic use of substances: An inductive model derived from a comparative analysis of the alcohol, opiate, tobacco, and food/obesity literatures. *International Journal of the Addictions*, *21*, 1–23.

Vaillant, G. E. (1973). A 20-year follow-up of New York narcotic addicts. *Archives of General Psychiatry*, *29*, 237–241.

Vaillant, G. E. (1983). *Natural history of alcoholism*. Cambridge, MA: Harvard University Press.

Waldorf, D., Reinarman, C., & Murphy, S. (1991). *Cocaine changes: The experience of using and quitting*. Philadelphia, PA: Temple University.

Weisner, C., Matzger, H., & Kaskutas, L. A. (2003). How important is treatment? One-year outcomes of treated and untreated alcohol-dependent individuals. *Addiction*, *98*(7), 901–911.

White, W. (2008). *Recovery management and recovery-oriented systems of care: Scientific rationale and promising practices*. Pittsburgh, PA: Northeast Addiction Technology Transfer Center, Great Lakes Addiction Technology Transfer Center, Philadelphia Department of Behavioral Health & Mental Retardation Services.

White, W., & Cloud, W. (2008). Recovery capital: A primer for addictions professionals. *Counselor*, *9*(5), 22–27.

White, W., & Kurtz, E. (2006). The varieties of recovery experience. *International Journal of Self-Help and Self-Care*, *3*(1/2), 21–61.

White, W., & Schulstad, M. (2009). Relapse following prolonged addiction recovery: Time for answers to critical questions. *Counselor*, *10*(4), 36–39.

Winick, C. (1962). Maturing out of narcotic addiction. *Bulletin on Narcotics*, *14*, 1–7.

A Discussion of the Origins of *The Road to Recovery*—the Scottish Government's Recovery Policy for Drugs

RIA DIN

Independent Adviser, Drugs & Alcohol, Glasgow, Scotland, United Kingdom

This article is an attempt to provide an overview of the origins of the Scottish Government's current drug strategy The Road to Recovery: A New Approach to Tackling Scotland's Drug Problem *(2008) and to provide an analysis of the particular national and local policymaking environment that shaped the strategy. Launched in May 2008, it signaled a paradigm change in thinking about drugs policy in relation to those with a serious drug problem in Scotland.*

OVERVIEW OF THE ORIGINS OF THE POLICY

This article is an attempt to provide an overview of the origins of the Scottish Government's current drug strategy *The Road to Recovery: A New Approach To Tackling Scotland's Drug Problem* (2008) and to provide an analysis of the particular national and local policymaking environment that shaped the strategy. Launched in May 2008, it signaled a paradigm change in thinking about drugs policy in relation to those with a serious drug problem in Scotland.

What led to this change in government policy, and why has it influenced the adoption of recovery as a way of understanding addictions and working with people in Scotland, and potentially in the rest of the United Kingdom?

Material for this article was gathered while Ria Din was on secondment as a specialist advisor in drugs to the Scottish Government between 2006 and 2011. The article is authored by Ria Din in a personal capacity and not as a representative of the Scottish Government.

The author would like to acknowledge the assistance of Dr. Maureen Bruce and Dr. Paul Bennett for their helpful suggestions on various drafts of this article.

Furthermore, how can we gauge, at the time of writing (November 2010) the progress of the policy in driving forward recovery as a working paradigm? Ultimately, and particularly in the run up to Scottish Government elections in 2011, government will be pressed to prove "recovery" as a policy work .

Although the previous policy, *Tackling Drugs in Scotland: Action in Partnership* (Scottish Office, 1999), aspired to many of the structural principles espoused in its successor, *Road to Recovery* (e.g., effective "partnership working"), it led to no measurable progress in being able to demonstrate the link between government policies and resources targeted at the issue and any accepted measure of "success."

As time for a successor to *Tackling Drugs in Scotland* drew nearer, a particular set of circumstances began to come together and led to the publication of a strategy signaling one of the most radical shifts in thinking on drugs policy published by a UK government in recent times.

In March 2007, the election of a new administration in Scotland allowed scope for a fresh look at drug policy. Before this could begin, the new Scottish Government wanted to take a fresh look itself at policymaking in general and its implementation.

SCOTLAND PERFORMS

The new Scottish Government established what it termed the "National Performance Framework," which aimed to enable all of those in the public sector to demonstrate what could be achieved with the total resources allocated to them. This would be done by using an "outcome-based" approach, measuring performance in what it achieved for the Scottish people across a range of indices, rather than in terms of outputs alone.

This approach was introduced with the first spending review of the new administration at the end of 2007.

The government itself described this new framework in the following terms:

> The National Performance Framework and outcome-based approach has an impact on every part of the [organization] (Scottish Government) and beyond. The framework will apply universally across the whole public sector, and will be used as a common basis for performance management. (Scottish Government, 2007)

In addition, the new Scottish Government sought to partner this approach with those working in a local context:

> The Scottish Government has a new 'Concordat' with local government in Scotland built on a mutual understanding and respect of each

others' roles, and a recognition that local government is best placed to understand and respond to local priorities, and they will link to the National Performance System through outcome agreements. (Scottish Government, 2009)

The Concordat also made clear that authorities would individually sign outcome agreements with national government, reflecting a [contextualized] focus on the national priorities. Local authorities would therefore be given new freedom to spend money, and to focus on those priorities that reflected local needs most directly, as long as they fed into the national purpose.

What this signaled was in fact a dramatic reform of public sector accountability all now linked to achievement of the National Performance Framework goals.

Together, the economic strategy, the Scottish Spending Review, and the National Performance Framework were all intended to fundamentally alter the relationship of the Scottish Government with local authorities.

It was in this context that *The Road to Recovery* was launched into a progressive strategy of delivering a new way of measuring performance linked to local need but which, it was hoped, would add up to a demonstrably better life for the people of Scotland.

The *Road to Recovery* also linked itself to the progressive social care agenda in the United Kingdom, such as the personalized care agenda and "self-directed care," both of which sought to empower the "end user" of services by allowing them to have a key role in deciding what they needed with the resources available to them.

DRUGS POLICY

Up until 2007 in Scotland at least, the public and press discourse on drugs could be generally categorized as reflecting the so-called "abstinence versus harm reduction debate." In the 15 years preceding the launch of *The Road to Recovery*, this had become shorthand for seemingly entrenched views on the "right" way to work with people with a drug problem. The early public health approaches of the 1980s, largely devised to tackle the rise for HIV, led to a largely "medicalized" approach to tackling the issue. The adoption of methadone maintenance as the core pillar of drug treatment by many National Health Service (NHS) and joint NHS/local authority service providers, and particularly in the community offender management system, became known as "the harm-reduction approach."—perhaps unfairly characterized as the polar opposite of this was the "abstinence approach." In reality, neither deserved to be considered mutually exclusive of the other, but this so-called "debate" left Scotland no further forward in tackling its growing drug problem. Neither approach appeared to be informed by the lived experience of people who had had a drug problem, and users or people in recovery seemed to be very much "passive recipients" of whatever policy and providers of services dictated (Scottish Government, 2008).

The new Scottish Government, noting the continued relentless press interest and ongoing public discussion about drugs misuse, as well as ever-present indicators of harm (e.g., drug-related deaths; General Registrars Office for Scotland, 2009), precipitated a number of investigations and reviews in the spring and summer of 2007:

- the publication of the "Methadone Review"—a review of methadone prescribing in Scotland instigated via the Scottish Advisory Committee on Drug Misuse (SACDM) by the previous government (SACDM: Methadone Project Group, 2007);
- the publication of a review of residential services, similarly commissioned by the previous administration; and
- a review of "essential care" (i.e., initially, those "services" required to help people come off and stay off drugs (SACDM: Integrated Care Project Group, 2008)

In addition, the Scottish Government funded a number of pilot projects to look at alternative ways of promoting recovery to the traditional treatment-based approach. One of these pilots in particular, the Lothians and Edinburgh Abstinence Program (LEAP) has gone on to be funded beyond the pilot stage. The Scottish Government also commissioned a review of LEAP (as yet unpublished; LEAP, 2010), which showed the effectiveness of its partnerships with residential and employability services to deliver recovery-focused outcomes for people using its service.

Concurrently, a process of "delivery reform," based on an earlier "stocktake" of alcohol and drug action teams (ADATs; Scottish Executive, 2007), was taking place and considering the effectiveness of the Drug Action Teams (DATS) or Alcohol and Drug Action Teams (ADATs) and their ability to deliver effective partnerships to tackle the national drug problem. Particularly in the light of newly established local community planning partnerships, this could be seen as a legitimate effort to make these partnerships (now to be known as alcohol and drug partnerships [ADPs]) both more effective and relevant to the new policy context (Alcohol and Drug Delivery Reform Group, 2009).

Discussions began on driving up standards of service provision, which were to lead to the development of a national NHS performance HEAT (Health Improvement, Efficiency, Access, Treatment) target to enable those with a serious drug problem to access assessments and then treatment within 3 weeks regardless of where in Scotland they lived. "HEAT" targets were seen as an effective part of the overarching "performance framework" (NHS Scotland, HEAT Performance Management Systems, 2010).

ESSENTIAL CARE

The working group to examine "essential care" became the main think tank that fed the development of a "recovery"-oriented drugs strategy within the Scottish Government. This group initially accepted that recovering from drug use was a process with much wider implications than anything that clinical treatment services only could offer.

At the same time, there was an enthusiasm within government for looking at other policy areas and being willing to learn from their experiences in trying to look afresh at seemingly entrenched approaches. The government's practice of drafting practitioners from the field to help influence policy also led to its openness to being influenced by other approaches put forward within government by these professional advisors. These influences had a direct bearing on introducing the concepts of recovery to those who were at that time instrumental in shaping policy within the government.

In terms of other policy "influences," one of these in particular—mental health policy—had embarked on a radical and exciting journey that led to the new mental health framework (Scottish Government, 2009).

This focused on the "recovery" of people with mental health problems and focused particularly on lessening stigma. Although not as advanced as the United States in making connections between the substance use and mental health agendas, connections were being made both within and beyond the Scottish Government between these two populations' lived experiences. At this stage, there were no direct links to, or indeed knowledge of, the emerging U.S. recovery movement heavily influenced by William White. These connections and influences were to subsequently become a significant part of recovery development in Scotland after the publication of the strategy.

In terms of both the mental health and learning disability experiences in the United Kingdom, approaches to these populations had themselves undergone massive paradigm shifts in thinking. Advocates of both approaches had worked in Scotland through the Scottish Recovery Network (mental health) and the Scottish Learning Disability Consortium to lessen stigma, build on people's strengths, and give people and their families a central place in directing their own care. Further than this, it sought to overcome narrow definitions of people by their label of patient or other stigmatizing and potentially limiting status and instead allow them the fullest possible potential as active and participating members of society with hope and aspirations like everyone else (Scottish Executive, 2001).

The challenge in drugs policy was no less significant. How could a message of hope and aspiration be applied here, how could people with a drug problem and all that potentially goes with it be seen as individuals who had strengths, who were entitled to have aspirations, and who did indeed have something to contribute to society?

Following the switch to an outcomes-based approach, the focus of policy development switched from outputs and inputs to consider "real outcomes for real people." When applied to people with an addiction problem, it rapidly became clear that recovery was to be the goal. If this was to be the case, then national policy was required to challenge the existing approach to one of thinking about drug addiction in these terms.

RECOVERY—THE NEW PARADIGM

As a paradigm, recovery had the advantage of not encouraging a polarization of opinion or of approach, such as the "harm reduction versus abstinence" debate. Recovery is a journey, individual to the person, and has a universal application. Everyone wants people with a serious drug problem to recover—what could be negative about this?

At the same time, the visibility of people in recovery was more evident. People were appearing at more and more residential and community rehabilitation "graduation ceremonies," generally because they had had access to treatment or had been encouraged to believe they could recover and were supported to do so. There were also reports that significant numbers of individuals had spontaneously recovered without going to treatment services (White & Kurtz, 2006). This evidence suggested that other factors were clearly at play in determining people's recovery, and not all of these were within the control of agencies or the government itself. Mutual aid groups, family, and community were and are playing a critical role in helping people to recover (Biernacki, 1986).

What focusing on recovery also did was promote a focus on an identity that transcended that of being a drug user or some of its more stigmatizing labels, with all their connotations of being worthless and marginalized. It sought to broaden the horizons of those in the field of drug treatment and drug users themselves from defining their identity by their problem. It did this by placing the focus on the person and giving them hope, by focusing on their strengths and linking them to all the other agencies, groups, and general resources of their community—helping them build "recovery capital" (Laudet & White, 2008).

In the new world, if the drugs treatment field supported by government had a role at all, it was about facilitating people's recovery by mirroring hope, by enabling them to feel recovery was possible, and by encouraging them to seize the opportunity to become a "normal" member of society, to have what they perceived everyone else to have, to be accepted, to be able to earn a living, to form stable relationships, to go on holiday, and to look like everyone else.

OPERATIONALIZING RECOVERY

Essentially, a recovery-oriented system of care (ROSC) or "recovery orientation" can be recognized by the following indicators, although this is not by any means an exhaustive list:

- Those in recovery are working in partnership with professionals and others where necessary to determine their own recovery journey.
- Where treatment is asked for, there is no sole mode of treatment but a variety of treatments or approaches on offer, all of them recovery focused.
- People in recovery are visible. Like any other user of public services, they are also visible in terms of their involvement and participation in the design and delivery of services—"nothing about us without us."
- It is recognized that recovery is not all about services, not all about more resources. People can be helped in a whole range of ways, not necessarily linked to formal treatment, which will help them to recover.

Although widely open to interpretation, recovery is an approach that can embrace everyone's idea of what that journey could be. It advocates neither abstinence nor maintenance but a future built around people's existing strengths where many things, including substitute prescribing, can help an individual achieve momentum on the road to recovery.

Attempts to co-opt the term recovery to mean abstinence have been largely dispelled, not least by the Scottish Government's own repeated insistence that recovery embraces all aspects of treatment and community resources, including—where it is the result of a joint decision by clinician and the individual in recovery—methadone.

Much progress has been made in trying to develop the necessary infrastructure to drive and support recovery. ADPs have now been established, many of which, with the help of Scottish Government "national support coordinators," have striven to genuinely understand and begin to implement ROSCs. They have now sought to incorporate ROSC's key principles into their thinking and practice.

GENERAL

Since the launch of the strategy, the new recovery paradigm has been largely embraced both by those in recovery and those working in the drugs treatment field. *The Road to Recovery* itself achieved cross-party support at its launch in 2008. This cross-party agreement was also echoed in the Scottish Parliament Drugs Debate in September 2010 (Scottish Parliament Web site, Parliamentary Transcripts). To date, there have been very few retreats to public or press "debates" of the "harm reduction versus abstinence" nature.

Progress has also been made by many NHS boards, both as partners within ADPs and on reducing assessment and treatment waiting times. Most now currently are on target to achieve a 3-week waiting time in all areas from referral to assessment by 2012.

However, the real challenge in relation to recovery is to now coordinate this strategic activity with recovery-oriented activity in communities and empower those in recovery themselves to take a lead and accumulate their own "recovery capital." It is also a significant challenge for recovery advocates, including the Scottish Government, to translate this type of discourse and the paradigm itself into the kind of language everyone can understand and own, and as importantly, into a practical vision of what recovery can achieve for individuals and communities.

EVIDENCE OF RECOVERY ACCEPTANCE AND MEASURING SUCCESS

Two years since the launch of *The Road to Recovery*, the Scottish Government is heartened by the evidence that the strategy is being embraced by those on the ground. Most notably:

- Many ADPs, with their newly established partnerships with community planning structures, are now working toward producing local strategies that are recovery focused and are actively involved in determining outcomes that are recovery focused. Many of them are linking with service users to ensure that their voices are heard.
- In these areas, recovery as an approach has been embraced, and work has begun on achieving culture change locally.
- The Scottish Drugs Recovery Consortium (SDRC) has been established and welcomed by the many individuals, agencies, ADPs, and others who wish to be partners and members. Its mission is to promote recovery and build capacity of individuals in recovery and communities to create the widest possible accepting environment for making recovery possible.
- Within communities and in partnership with voluntary and statutory agencies, the "recovery café" (Kuladharini, 2010) movement is taking hold and providing informal one-off or regular events where those experiencing recovery or wishing to spread its message can share ideas and inspiration and pass on that knowledge and experience to new members.
- There is genuine growth of people in recovery becoming involved in organizing recovery events such as this autumn's Recovery Walk in Scotland (SDRC Newsletter, 2010)

- There is also an increase in the sharing of narrative experiences online, in written form, and in person, which provide hope and inspiration to those seeking recovery.

RESEARCH FOR RECOVERY

The publication of *Research for Recovery* in September 2010 (Best, Rome, Hanning, & White, 2010), commissioned by the Scottish Government, established that:

- The evidence base on recovery is growing and demonstrates that recovery-focused approaches can augment and enhance standard treatment approaches and maximize wider benefits to families and communities.
- The recovery journey typically lasts 5 to 7 years (to get former problem drug users to the point where they are no more likely to take illicit drugs than the general population).

Findings from this review emphasize:

- the importance of providing ongoing support to individuals following structured treatment;
- the positive outcomes associated with mutual aid and peer support in the community; and
- the importance of assertive (proactive) follow-up support.

It is intended that this will provide a springboard for establishing a solid framework for gathering evidence of how recovery as a strategy and as a policy is working for the people of Scotland affected by drugs misuse.

Ultimately, the success of the policy will be judged by the Scottish Government and others' ability to report progress on recovery-oriented outcomes in a way that is meaningful and credible. No doubt it will also come down to whether or not it can be demonstrated that as a result of the policy on recovery being established in practice and executed well, fewer people are using drugs or going on to problematic use. However, links to other outcome measurements must also be included.

If we are serious about viewing people who have had a drug problem as members of communities like everyone else, then we must judge their progress as we would any other member of those communities, by improved health, social well-being, and improved economic status. In this sense, the Scottish Government will encourage the gathering of evidence of improved outcomes for those affected by serious drug use, linked to the National Performance Framework, and through single outcome agreements, as agreed for all of the work of the Scottish Government and its partners locally.

Critical to this review of outcomes, however, must be the lived experience of those in recovery, as well as those affected by it, such as families and communities.

The greatest demonstration of *The Road to Recovery*'s success will be the increasing and highly visible presence of those in recovery themselves, making their own longed-for contribution to society and demonstrating that there is hope and that recovery is in fact possible. That will indeed continue to be a cause for celebration.

REFERENCES

Alcohol and Drug Delivery Reform Group. (2009). *Report of the Alcohol and Drug Delivery Reform Group*. Edinburgh, Scotland: Scottish Government.

Best, D., Rome, K, Hanning, A., & White, W. (2010). *Research for recovery: A review of the drugs evidence base/A review of international evidence to support Scotland's national drugs strategy, the road to recovery*. Retrieved from http://www.scotland.gov.uk/Publications/2010/08/18112230/16

Biernacki, P. (1986). *Pathways from heroin addiction without Treatment*. Philadelphia, PA: Temple University Press.

General Registrars Office for Scotland. (2009). *Drug-related deaths in Scotland*. Retrieved from http://www.gro-scotland.gov.uk/statistics/theme/vital-events/deaths/drug-related/drd2009/index.html

Kuladharini. (2009, December 12). Recovery conversation café—to go! A viral approach to peer influencing. *Wired In to Recovery*. [Web log]. Retrieved from http://wiredin.org.uk/blogs/entry/5930/recovery-conversation-cafe-to-go-a-viral-approach-to-peer-influencing/

Laudet, A. B., & White, W. L. (2008). Recovery capital as prospective predictor of sustained recovery, life satisfaction, and stress among former polysubstance users. *Substance Use and Misuse, 43*(1), 27–54.

The Lothians and Edinburgh Abstinence Program. (2010). *Scottish Government commissioned research*. Unpublished report.

NHS Scotland, HEAT Performance Management Systems. (2010, April). Target A11 to offer drug misusers faster access to appropriate treatment to support their recovery. Retrieved from http://www.scotland.gov.uk/Topics/Justice/law/Drugs-Strategy/recovery/HEAT/referral-pathways

Scottish Advisory Committee on Drug Misuse: Integrated Care Project Group. (2008). *Essential care: A report on the approach required to maximize opportunity for recovery from problem substance use in Scotland*. Edinburgh, Scotland: Scottish Government.

Scottish Advisory Committee on Drug Misuse: Methadone Project Group. (2007). *Reducing harm and promoting recovery: A report on methadone treatment for substance misuse in Scotland*. Edinburgh, Scotland: Scottish Government.

Scottish Executive. (2001). *The same as you: A review of services for people with learning disabilities*. Retrieved from http://www.scotland.gov.uk/Resource/Doc/159140/0043285.pdf

Scottish Executive. (2007). *Report of the stocktake of alcohol and drug action teams.* Retrieved from http://www.scotland.gov.uk/Publications/2007/06/22094551/0

Scottish Government. (2009, May). *Toward a mentally flourishing Scotland: The future of mental health improvement in Scotland 2008–11.* Retrieved from http://www.scotland.gov.uk/Publications/2007/10/26112853/1

Scottish Government. (2008). *The road to recovery: A new approach to tackling Scotland's drug problem.* Edinburgh, Scotland: Author.

Scottish Government. (2007, November). Scottish Government budget review. Retrieved from http://www.scotland.gov.uk/Publications/2007/11/13092240/0

Scottish Government. (2009, March). *In the line of sight.* National School of Government. Retrieved from http://virtual.nationalschool.gov.uk/StrategyExchange/Documents/Scotland%20final.pdf

Scottish Office. (1999). *Tackling drugs in Scotland: Action in partnership.* Retrieved from http://www.scotland.gov.uk/Resource/Doc/158170/0042803.pdf.

Scottish Parliament. (2010, September 15). *Official report 15 September 2010.* Retrieved from http://www.scottish.parliament.uk/business/officialreports/meetingsparliament/or-10/sor0915-02.htm

White, W., & Kurtz E.. (2006). *Linking addiction treatment and communities of recovery: A primer for addiction counselors and recovery coaches.* Pittsburgh, PA: IRETA. Retrieved from http://store.ireta.org/merchant2/merchant.mvc?Screen=PROD&Store_Code=I&Product_Code=mng995-DLD1.zip&Category_Code=mng

North West Recovery Forum: Recovery and Harm Reduction, the Odd Couple of Drug Treatment?

MARK GILMAN

North West Regional Manager, National Treatment for Substance Abuse, Manchester, England, United Kingdom

ROWDY YATES

Scottish Addiction Studies, Department of Applied Social Sciences, University of Stirling, Stirling, Scotland, United Kingdom

Harm reduction and recovery are not mutually exclusive concepts, and it is perfectly possible to build a recovery orientation into or onto an existing harm-reduction-oriented treatment structure. This short article chronicles the work of the North West Recovery Forum in England in bringing together treatment providers and purchasers, community activists, international recovery experts, and people in recovery to move treatment services toward a recovery vision and grow recovery-friendly communities.

INTRODUCTION

For almost three decades, substitute prescribing (most often, methadone maintenance treatment [MMT]), within the context of a harm-reduction paradigm, has been the dominant treatment intervention in the United Kingdom. Initially, this change of direction in UK drug policy was triggered by concerns over the infection potential of needle-sharing drug users (Yates, 2002) with the emergence of HIV/AIDS. More latterly, the dominance of a treatment response essentially predicated upon containment and management of the problem has been further sustained by concerns over the apparent relationship between drug misuse and crime.

However, containment and resolution of a problem—or in this case, harm reduction and recovery—are not mutually oppositional concepts. Indeed, recovery-oriented interventions, like harm reduction, can deliver significant societal gains in both infection control and crime reduction.

In recent years, there has been a significant rebirth of interest in recovery as a central element in our treatment response (Ashton, 2008; Yates & Malloch, 2010). Much of this has been inspired by, and driven by, service users themselves, although, perhaps inevitably, the issue has become a profoundly political one (Ashton, 2008). Best and colleagues (2010) have argued that the resistance to change within the treatment field has misinterpreted the nature of the change and largely overlooked the evidence base for recovery.

This short article chronicles the coming together in the North West of England of a number of networks and organizations to explore the possibility of building a recovery orientation onto an existing model of harm reduction and substitute prescribing. It argues that not only is such a development eminently possible but that it is critical for the long-term efficacy of mainstream treatment structures.

HISTORICAL CONTEXT

The North West of England is dominated by the conurbations of Merseyside and Greater Manchester. The home of the industrial revolution was also home to the first wave of brown powder heroin that arrived in the United Kingdom in the early 1980s (Pearson, Gilman, & McIver, 1985). Many of the working-class users of heroin began by smoking the drug. As they became dependent on heroin, they switched to injecting for economic reasons, because a bag of heroin that is injected represents better value for money (Pearson & Gilman, 2005). However, an injection heroin addiction cannot be paid for out of an ordinary working-class wage or welfare payment. Consequently, acquisitive crime rose alongside the rise in the number of heroin addicts (Parker, Bakx, & Newcombe, 1988).

By 1986, the North West of England drug treatment systems were faced with a public health and crime prevention challenge. Harm reduction emerged as the solution to prevent the spread of HIV from injecting drug users to the wider population and to reduce acquisitive crime (McDermott, 2005). Harm reduction policy saw the introduction of needle and syringe distribution and exchange programs and the widespread provision of opioid substitute medication on a maintenance basis. The expansion in the provision of opioid substitute medication on a maintenance basis was prompted and supported by a variety of influential interest groups. The police supported MMT because it reduced crime. Ward, Mattick, and Hall (1992) have argued that criminal behavior halves with each year that a patient remains in treatment. The UK's National Probation Service supported MMT for this same reason. Namely, it reduces criminal behavior and can therefore keep people out of prison (Gilman & Pearson, 1991). Public health professionals supported MMT because "being in methadone treatment has been associated with lower rates of HIV infection for opiate injectors than not being in treatment" (Ward et al., p. 61). Doctors support MMT because it prevents opiate overdose and death (Caplehorn, Stellay, Dalton, Cluff, & Petrenas, 1994). MMT also has support among some patient advocacy groups such as the Methadone Alliance (subsequently, simply "The Alliance"; Joyce, 2010).

In essence, the expansion in MMT was due to the evidence that it kept opioid-dependent people alive and out of prison. Moreover, it appeared to be able to do so economically. In the world of UK health care systems, methadone, as a medication, is not an expensive option. Currently, MMT can be purchased and provided for approximately £2,000 per patient per year. To put this into perspective, a commissioner could purchase 10 annual MMT "slots" for the price of one "slot" in a traditional inpatient withdrawal and residential rehabilitation program. However, it should be noted that this apparent saving may be largely chimeral. Some commentators (Berg & Andersen, 1993; French, Sacks, De Leon, Staines, & McKendrick, 1999; Unell & Vincent, 1994; Yates, 2010) have argued that when like is genuinely compared to like and the evaluative timeframe takes adequate account of posttreatment cost benefits, residential treatment may be significantly cheaper.

The funding for harm reduction interventions and treatment continued throughout the 1980s, 1990s, and 2000s. Public expenditure on drug and alcohol treatment is notoriously difficult to estimate, and expenditure within the private sector is effectively unknown. The UK Government, in its annual report to the European Monitoring Center for Drugs and Drugs Addiction, estimates "labeled" expenditure for 2007–2008 at slightly below £1 billion (Eaton et al., 2008). However, this figure is calculated using the United Nations Classification of Functions of Government and excludes a number of significant funding streams. Similarly, the UK Government's most recent strategy document (HM Government, 2008), *Drugs: Protecting Families and Communities*, estimates "labeled" expenditure at £958 million for 2009–2010 but notes that around £1.2 billion will be spent in related areas. A more extensive calculation of Scottish public sector expenditure on alcohol and drugs has been undertaken by Audit Scotland (2009). This estimates total expenditure at £173 million, with around 68% of this being invested in treatment services.[1] For the United Kingdom as a whole, the Royal Society for the Arts (2006) has estimated that the percentage of total "labeled" expenditure allocated to treatment hovers around 38% to 40%, while the percentage for research and evaluation is less than 1%.

Whatever the true costs of UK public spending in addiction treatment services, it would appear undeniable, that significant funding is being invested and that this funding has increased dramatically in real terms in the past two decades (Ashton, 2008). By 2010, the total investment was close to

£1 billion. The success of this investment is seen primarily in the control of HIV and the prevention of drug-related acquisitive crime. The public health and public safety model of harm reduction continues to deliver societal benefit and is supported by the general public (National Treatment Agency, 2009). This model requires treatment and intervention systems to do three things: firstly, to make contact with injection drug users via needle and syringe programs; secondly, to maintain contact with those same people via the provision of opioid substitution medication on a maintenance basis; and thirdly, to effect change (Ashton & Seymour, 1988; Lowell & Ashton, 2007). Thus, the emergence of the recovery agenda in the North West of England in 2005 can be seen as the implementation of the third phase of a process that began in 1986. Recovery is about making change. In 2005, the North West had a large and efficient treatment system that processed 35,469 people with substance use disorders (Khundakar, Marr, McVeigh, & Bellis, 2006). It was easy for service users to get into the system ("access") and easy for them to stay in ("retention"). Leaving the medical treatment system and engaging with the social world of recovery have proven more challenging. The North West Recovery Forum was established in 2005 to meet that challenge and establish recovery-oriented integrated systems (Gilman & Yates, 2010).

ORGANIZATIONAL CONTEXT

The North West is one of nine regions in England for the funding of drug treatment. There are 22 local authorities or councils in the North West of England. Each of these has a local strategic partnership (LSP). This is a single body that brings together at a local level the different parts of the public sector, as well as the private, business, community, and voluntary sectors, so that different initiatives and services support each other and work together. The LSP is a nonstatutory partnership. It provides a single overarching local coordination framework within which other partnerships can operate (Audit Commission, 2009). It is responsible for developing and driving the implementation of community strategies and local area agreements (LAAs). One of the strategic drivers for the North West Recovery Forum was the emergence of LAAs and the interest of LSPs in the drug treatment agenda. The drug treatment effort in Liverpool and Manchester and the 20 other areas in the North West is the responsibility of the drug and alcohol action teams in each of those areas. In theory, the DAATs operate under the umbrella of—or at least link to—the LSP (McGrail & MacKintosh, 2008). In practice, the DAATs have tended to operate without reference to their relevant LSP and in many cases have become local independent bureaucracies collating and providing performance management data on drug treatment directly to English regional and central government. In the construction of LAAs, the drug treatment effort was included by way of an indicator of the numbers of problematic drug users in effective treatment. The working assumption was that increasing the numbers in effective treatment would contribute to public health, crime reduction, and community safety.

In August 2005, Blackburn with Darwen Council (one of the 22 in the North West) had a meeting of its LSP and discussed drug treatment. The Blackburn with Darwen LSP and Public Service Board asked a simple question: "Drug treatment in Blackburn: Is it any good?" Most of the discussion centered on aspiration and ambition. LSP members wondered whether drug treatment could do more than "keep people alive and out of jail" (Best, 2010, p. 33). LSP members wanted to know if drug treatment could play a role in addressing "worklessness." At that time, worklessness was a "big ticket item" in Blackburn with Darwen. There was much concern about people who were chemically dependent on substances and financially dependent on welfare payments. Many of these people were registered unable to work as a result of being incapacitated or disabled by their substance use disorders. LSP members wanted to know if treatment could be improved or enhanced so that substance use disorders could be treated in such a way as to ensure that people could become abstinent, enter employment, training, or education, and leave the lifestyle of welfare dependency behind.

They asked also whether drug treatment could be expected to equip parents to care for their own children. Many of those with substance use disorders are also in very poor physical and mental health. There are a large number of children in the North West who have to be looked after by the local authority because of parental substance use disorders and/or poor physical/mental health. LSP members wondered whether improved drug treatment could play a role in addressing the stark health inequalities in the borough, which appeared to coexist alongside these incidents of "looked-after children."

Most challenging of all was the question of whether improved drug treatment could be expected to prevent the intergenerational transmission of substance use disorders.

The answer to all these questions was that substance use disorder treatment *could* be expected to address all of these big ticket items *if* the treatment system had a recovery orientation. However, it could not be expected to address these issues if the treatment system revolved around the provision of symptomatic medical relief in the shape of opioid substitution medication on a maintenance basis, with little else provided of greater ambition. In short, the treatment system had to move from the medical to the social. But it had to do this without losing the public health and safety gains made during the previous 20 years. It was decided that the best way of modernizing and improving drug treatment would be to move to a recovery orientation by entering into a consultation process with members of the North West Recovery Forum.

BUILDING THE RECOVERY BRIDGE FROM MEDICAL TO SOCIAL

Stuart Honor and his colleagues have been investigating the social reality of drug treatment for the past decade (Honor, 2006). Using qualitative methods of social inquiry, their work consistently challenges the view of the world derived via orthodox medical research on the role of treatment in the lives of addicts. Honor's work is in the tradition of Preble and Casey (1969), Johnson, Williams, Dei, and Sanabria (1990), and Bourgois (1996) and shows the role that a drug like methadone plays in the everyday lives of welfare-dependent addicts. His work also shows that polydrug use is now the norm across the North West of England. Crack cocaine, alcohol, and benzodiazepines often feature in the daily using patterns of addicts in and out of maintenance substitute medication programs. Honor is a founding member of the North West Recovery Forum, and his work has consistently carried the message that treatment needs to modernize, improve, and embrace recovery.

The problem for treatment providers who agreed with the message was in understanding how this might be achieved. To this end, members of the North West Recovery Forum (who were not themselves in recovery) attended open meetings of 12-step mutual aid groups (Alcoholics Anonymous, Narcotics Anonymous, and Cocaine Anonymous) and alumni meetings of residential rehabilitation treatment providers. Self-Management and Recovery Training (SMART) Recovery meetings also welcomed members of the North West Recovery Forum. The practical lesson was clear. Substance use disorder may be a chronic condition that is characterized by relapse (McLellan, Lewis, O'Brien, & Kleber, 2000), but it is also a condition that people recover from. Many millions have recovered by following the 12 steps as set out in the *Big Book* of Alcoholics Anonymous in the 1930s (Alcoholics Anonymous, 2002). Service managers must insist that anyone working in the treatment of substance use disorders can demonstrate a thorough knowledge and understanding of the workings of mutual aid recovery groups.

Honor's (2006) work shows us that there are many addicts still suffering in treatment and desperate to hear the message of experience, strength, and hope offered by a fellow addict in recovery. Where this is working well, people with a substance use disorder are encouraged by the treatment community to move into the "circles of recovery" (Humphreys, 2004). If recovery proves too much of a challenge, then people can go back onto substitute medication and reflect on their experiences of recovery. They will always be welcomed back into the circles of recovery when they are ready to try again. In time, recovery in treatment on substitute opioid treatment may become a reality. This will happen when significant numbers of people in medical substitute medication-based treatment are off welfare, employed, and looking after their own children in their own homes.

RECOVERY COMMUNITIES

Recovery in individuals begins with the practical alleviation of the physical symptoms of dependency. For those on a recovery journey to abstinence, this involves physical withdrawal. Depending on personal circumstance and access to resources, this can be done in the community or as an inpatient. Either way, detoxification has always been the easy part. Getting off is easy; staying off is hard. That is why some kind of psychosocial intervention is required. In the North West, treatment providers have been involved in the improvement of psychosocial interventions by way of our involvement with the International Treatment Effectiveness Project (ITEP). This began in 2005 and is ongoing (Simpson, 2009).

The recurring themes of ITEP are journeys and maps. Routes and pathways from active addiction to treatment to recovery are increasing. Those who have trodden those paths and those who have helped them have gained extensive experience that is shared with people starting out on their own journeys. ITEP is all about movement, dynamism, journeys, and maps of optimism. This stands in stark contrast to the stagnation and apparent pessimism of the orthodox medical treatment that we set out to change (Gilman, 2010). People change. People get off substances. People address their psychosocial conditions. People map their own routes to recovery. However, we humans are social animals. We do not do this alone. All along the way, we are interacting with other humans. Somewhere down the road of recovery, we start to address environmental issues.

The North West of England used to invest significant sums of money in sending people with substance use disorders away from the North West for residential treatments. Those who did well usually stayed away and did not return to the North West. Many of the North West's residential rehabilitation successes were enjoyed by communities outside our region. Those who had relapsed came back to the North West and told commissioners that residential rehabilitation had not worked. Commissioners started to wonder about the value for money proposition of residential rehabilitation. The reason that people who had done well did not return to the North West is because the environments to which they were returning were not recovery friendly. In fact, it could be argued that they were actively hostile to recovery. It soon became clear that we needed to think about "indigenous recovery" and recovery communities in the North West. We wanted people to believe that they could "get well where they got sick."

This belief is very hard if you have never met anyone who has done it. If all you know about treatment is the kind of world described by Honor

(2006) and colleagues, then the very idea of recovery can seem idealistic. In this arena, we were supported by, and are indebted to, our colleagues and partners in the United States. William White (2010) introduced us to Dr. Arthur Evans and colleagues in Philadelphia and to Phil Valentine and colleagues in Connecticut. Obviously, the United Kingdom and the United States are very different for all kinds of reasons (not least our welfare state). However, we found that our differences on the recovery community agenda were few. We had much more in common than we could have imagined. When harm reduction was the key organizing principle for drug treatment systems, many UK treatment "experts" established partnerships with colleagues in Europe (O'Hare, Newcombe, Matthews, Buning, & Drucker, 1992). In an era dominated by recovery, UK treatment "experts" are busily establishing partnerships with colleagues in the United States. Treatment contracts in excess of £6 million are being won and lost in the North West on the basis of the provider's proposals to embrace recovery. The North West Recovery Forum is building a bridge that unites recovery and treatment. Similar construction projects are underway all over the United Kingdom.

CONCLUSION

Harm reduction-based interventions have dominated the treatment of substance use disorder in England for 25 years. The benefits of harm reduction have been primarily societal. Drug-driven crime and the transmission of HIV have been reduced and prevented. The North West Recovery forum values these gains and seeks to build on them. International, national, regional, and local recovery forums are seeking to bring individuals and communities back into the picture. Recovery from substance misuse disorders in individuals spreads out from the physical to the environmental. The first stage involves addressing the physical symptoms of dependence (e.g., detoxification). The second stage involves an exploration of the psychological problems that are involved in substance use disorders. The third stage involves repairing relationships with family and friends. The fourth stage involves the environment, community, and society. At some point in this process, people in recovery have the potential to become an asset in community development. Recovery forums need to join forces with others involved in forms of asset-based community development (Kretzman, McKnight, Dobrowolski, & Puntenney, 2005). In the North West of England, addiction to heroin spread from one vulnerable person to another via friendship networks. Addiction to heroin became polydrug use and is rooted in the most vulnerable people in the most vulnerable families in the most vulnerable communities. The North West Recovery Forum has brought together all those who have a stake in recovery and has become as contagious as addiction. Our social networks have a fundamental influence on the shape of our lives. We are all connected (Christakis & Fowler, 2009). Members of recovery forums are engaged in producing the tipping point from addiction to recovery (Gladwell, 2001) at the community and societal levels.

NOTE

1. By population size, Scotland is roughly 10% of the UK total, although, due to differing demographics, this is not necessarily accurately reflected in overall expenditure.

REFERENCES

Alcoholics Anonymous. (2002). *Alcoholics Anonymous: The big book* (4th ed.). Center City, MN: Hazelden Information & Educational Services.

Ashton, M. (2008, December/January). The new abstentionists. *Druglink* (Special Insert). Retrieved from http://www.drugscope.org.uk/Resources/ Drugscope/Documents/PDF/Good%20Practice/Ashton_M_30.pdf

Ashton, J., & Seymour, H. (1988). *The new public health: The Liverpool experience.* Milton Keynes, UK: Open University Press.

Audit Commission. (2009). *Working better together? Managing local strategic partnerships.* London, UK: Author.

Audit Scotland. (2009). *Drug and alcohol services in Scotland.* Edinburgh, Scotland: Author.

Berg, J., & Andersen, S. (1993). Drug addict rehabilitation: A burden on society. *International Journal of Rehabilitation Research, 15,* 301–309.

Best, D. (2010). Mapping routes to recovery: The role of recovery groups and communities. In R. Yates & M. Malloch (Eds.), *Tackling addiction: Pathways to recovery* (pp. 32–43). London, UK: Jessica Kingsley.

Best, D., Bamber, S., Battersby, A., Gilman, M., Groshkova, T., Honor, S., . . . White, W. (2010). Recovery and straw men: An analysis of the objections raised to the transition to a recovery model in UK addiction services. *Journal of Groups in Addiction & Recovery, 5,* 264–288.

Bourgois, P. (1996). *In search of respect: Selling crack in El Barrio.* Cambridge, UK: Cambridge University Press.

Caplehorn, J., Stellay, M., Dalton, N., Cluff, M., & Petrenas, A. (1994). Retention in methadone maintenance and heroin addicts' risk of death. *Addiction, 89,* 203–207.

Christakis, N. A., & Fowler, J. H. (2009). *Connected: The surprising power of our social networks and how they shape our lives.* New York, NY: Little & Brown.

Eaton, G., Davies, C., English, L., Lodwick, A., McVeigh, J., & Bellis, M. (2008). *United Kingdom focal point report 2008.* Lisbon, Portugal: UK Focal Point/European Monitoring Center for Drugs and Drugs Addiction.

French, M. T., Sacks, S., De Leon, G., Staines, G., & McKendrick, K. (1999). Modified therapeutic community for mentally ill chemical abusers: Outcomes and costs. *Evaluation and the Health Professions, 22,* 60–85.

Gilman, M. (2010). *Once upon a time in the North West: Challenging the drug treatment system in England* [DVD]. Liverpool, UK: Genie in the Gutter.

Gilman, M., & Pearson, G. (1991). Lifestyles and law enforcement. In D. K. Whines & P. T. Bean (Eds.), *Policing and prescribing* (pp. 95–124). London, UK: Macmillan.

Gilman, M., & Yates, R. (2010). NW ROIS: Recovery-oriented integrated systems in North West England. In R. Yates & M. Malloch (Eds.), *Tackling addiction: Pathways to recovery* (pp. 84–95). London, UK: Jessica Kingsley.

Gladwell, M. (2001). *The tipping point*. London, UK: Little, Brown Book Group.

HM Government. (2008). *Drugs: Protecting families and communities*. London, UK: Her Majesty's Stationery Office (HMSO).

Honor, S. (2006). *Breaking glass: Problem drug use in St Helens*. St. Helens, UK: Baseline Research and Development.

Humphreys, K. (2004). *Circles of recovery: Self-help organizations for addictions*. Cambridge, UK: Cambridge University Press.

Johnson, B. D., Williams, T., Dei, K., & Sanabria, H. (1990). Drug abuse in the inner city: Impact on hard drug users and the community. In M. Tonry & J. Q. Wilson (Eds.), *Drugs and crime* (pp. 9–67). Chicago, IL; London, UK: University of Chicago Press.

Joyce, A. (2010, May 24). Talking heads. *Drink and Drugs News*, p. 10. Retrieved from http://www.drinkanddrugsnews.com/magazine/491c569c98d04758af2ab 107f168342f.pdf

Khundakar, A., Marr, A., McVeigh, J., & Bellis, M. (2006). *Drug treatment in the North West of England*. Liverpool, UK: Center for Public Health, John Moores University.

Kretzman, J. P., McKnight, J. L., Dobrowolski, S., & Puntenney, D. (2005). *Discovering community power: A guide to mobilizing local assets and your organization's capacity*. Evanston, IL: ABCD Institute, Northwestern University.

Lowell, L., & Ashton, J. (2007). Starting where they are is the key to providing for underserved groups. *Journal of Epidemiology and Community Health*, *61*, 27.

McDermott, P. (2005). The great Mersey experiment: The birth of harm reduction. In J. Strang and M. Gossop (Eds.), *Heroin addiction and the British system* (Vol. 1, pp. 122–136). Abingdon, NY: Routledge.

McGrail, S., & MacKintosh, D. (2008). *The national drug strategy: A guide for local partnerships*. London, UK: London Drug Policy Forum.

McLellan, A. T., Lewis, D. C., O'Brien, C. P., & Kleber, H. D. (2000). Drug dependence, a chronic medical illness: Implications for treatment, insurance, and outcomes evaluation. *Journal of the American Medical Association*, *284*, 1689–1695.

National Treatment Agency. (2009, December 14). *Public value drug treatment because it makes their communities safer and reduces crime* [Press release].

O'Hare, P., Newcombe, R., Matthews, A., Buning, E., & Drucker, E. (Eds.). (1992). *The reduction of drug-related harm*. London, UK: Routledge.

Parker, H., Bakx, K., & Newcombe, R. (1988). *Living with heroin: The impact of a drugs 'epidemic' on an English community*. Milton Keynes, UK: Open University Press.

Pearson, G., & Gilman, M. (2005). Drug epidemics in space and time: Local diversity, subcultures, and social exclusion. In J. Strang & M. Gossop (Eds.),

Heroin addiction and the British system (Vol. 1, pp. 91–107). Abingdon, NY: Routledge.

Pearson, G., Gilman M., & McIver, S. (1985). *Young people and heroin: An examination of heroin use in the North of England.* London, UK: Health Education Council.

Preble, E., & Casey, J. J. (1969). Taking care of business: The heroin user's life on the street. *International Journal of the Addictions, 4,* 1–24.

Royal Society for the Arts. (2006). *The economic impact of illegal drug use* (Discussion Document). London, UK: Author.

Simpson, D. (2009). *Adaptation and implementation of TCU mapping: Enhanced counseling and assessment resources in the UK* (Institute of Behavioral Research Technical Report). Fort Worth, TX: Texas Christian University.

Unell, I., & Vincent, J. (1994). *The costs of residential care and services in the community for problem users of drugs and alcohol.* Loughborough, UK: Loughborough University of Technology.

Ward, J., Mattick, R., & Hall, W. (1992). *Key issues in methadone maintenance treatment.* Sydney, Australia: New South Wales University Press.

White, W. L. (2010). *The selected papers of William L. White: 1969 to present.* Retrieved from http://www.williamwhitepapers.com

Yates, R. (1999). Only available in black: The limiting of addiction services in the 20th century. In *Uteseksjonen 30 Ar Pa Gata, November 1999.* Oslo, Norway: Uteseksjonen. http://www.drugslibrary.stir.ac.uk/documents/black.pdf

Yates, R. (2002). A brief history of British drug policy, 1950–2001. *Drugs, Education, Prevention, and Policy, 9,* 113–124.

Yates, R. (2010). Recovery we can afford: An analysis of a sample of comparative cost-based studies. *International Journal of Therapeutic Communities, 31*(2), 145–156.

Yates, R., & Malloch, M. (2010). The road less traveled? A short history of addiction recovery. In R. Yates & M. Malloch (Eds.), *Tackling addiction: Pathways to recovery* (pp. 15–31). London, UK: Jessica Kingsley.

LEAP and the Recovery Community in Edinburgh

DAVID McCARTNEY

Lothians & Edinburgh Abstinence Program, Edinburgh, Scotland, United Kingdom

The Lothians and Edinburgh Abstinence Program is a quasiresidential integrated treatment program for patients in the Lothian area wanting to achieve abstinent recovery. The program was commissioned as a Scottish Government pilot project and is delivered through the health service. A partnership between health, housing, education, and employability services, the program incorporates the assets already existing in the recovery community locally to help patients sustain their recoveries after treatment. Taking a narrative approach, this article explores the context in which the service is set and its origins, development, and evolution and examines its relationship with local recovery communities. Learning from these experiences is detailed.

SCOTTISH CONTEXT

Scotland has a population of just over 5 million people. It has a national government that has powers devolved to it by UK government, including the areas of health and criminal justice. It is estimated that there are more than 55,000 problem drug users in Scotland corresponding to the 1.6% of the population aged 15 to 64 years old (Hay, Gannon, Casey, & McKeganey, 2009). This is higher than the estimated prevalence in England. It is amongst the highest in Europe.

Policy to deal with the problem has evolved over the years since the heroin "epidemic" of the 1980s. Initially, this was fueled by public health concerns around containing the spread of the HIV. When the National Treatment

Outcome Research Study (NTORS) was published (Gossop et al., 1997), it showed significant reductions in crime for problem opiate users in treatment with methadone in England. An estimate was made that for every pound spent on treatment, three pounds were saved from reduction in crime alone. As a result, a rapid expansion of methadone maintenance treatment facilities throughout the United Kingdom ensued and crime reduction attained a higher priority. Scotland's approach today remains a medically dominated model with prescribing at its heart, although there is now evidence of a change of direction driven by a new government policy.

The Drug Outcome Research in Scotland study (DORIS) revealed in 2004 that a majority of problem drug users coming to treatment set abstinence as a goal, but that most received harm reduction or maintenance treatment (McKeganey, Morris, Neale, & Robertson, 2004). The authors called for harm reduction services to "be assiduous in explaining to clients the reason for their focus and for ensuring that drug users have access to an array of services," including those that "are more oriented towards abstinence" (p. 423).

In Scotland, it is estimated that 22,000 people are currently receiving methadone maintenance treatment (Scottish Government, 2007, p. 2), but it is not known how many clients with problem drug use move on to abstinence from methadone or what proportion of those coming for help access treatment focused on recovery. There is of yet little awareness of "maintained recovery," and research from England (Best, Groshkova, & McTague, 2009) suggests that in some maintenance settings there is effectively little, if any, therapeutic input.

The DORIS study in its 3-year outcomes found that those achieving abstinence improved across a range of outcomes compared with those who were maintained on prescription opiates. The study also found that those recruited from residential treatment settings achieved abstinence at three times the rate of those in community treatment programs and five times the rate of those in prison-based treatment (McKeganey, Bloor, Robertson, Neale, & MacDougall, 2006). As the authors acknowledge, the nature of a cohort study makes the attribution of causality problematic. The DORIS study impacted little on treatment approaches. In England, the evidence from the NTORS study (Gossop et al., 1997) did influence policy and played a part in shaping the *Models of Care* policy document (National Treatment Agency [NTA], 2002).

In a 2004 review (Griesbach, et al., 2004), the Scottish Executive estimated that there were 21 detoxification and residential rehabilitation units in Scotland offering a total of 329 beds. In 2003 to 2004, an estimated 1,294 patients were admitted to those beds. The report also makes the point that some areas elected not to send any clients to residential treatment on the basis of cost and of being unconvinced of efficacy. McKeganey et al. (2006) report that only 2% of those coming to treatment services access residential rehabilitation. According to the NTA, low rates of access to residential treatment also existed in England (Best, O'Grady, Charalampous, & Gordon, 2005).

The Scottish Government asked their specialist advisory group, the Scottish Advisory Committee on Drug Misuse (SACDM), to commission a report on methadone prescribing in Scotland. This was published in 2007 and recommended that methadone remain the central plank of treatment for problem opiate use (SACDM Methadone Project Group, 2007). However, it also found that methadone could not be the whole solution, that there was a significant lack of services that would allow people to recover, and that there was a significant lack of information about outcomes from existing services. A further report was commissioned and published and found, among other things, that a wider range of nonmedical aspects of care were required, that a person-centered approach was preferable, that recovery must become the focus of care above treatment type and that problem substance users were entitled to the same quality of care as other patients (SACDM, 2008).

SCOTTISH DRUGS STRATEGY

Partly based on these reports, in 2008, the Scottish Government published its new drug strategy, *The Road to Recovery: A New Approach to Tackling Scotland's Drug Problem*. This set "recovery" as the specific aim of treatment and determined that a range of treatment and rehabilitation services ought to be available and that treatment services needed to integrate with generic services to fully address all the needs of those in treatment and not just their addiction. A further challenge to those tasked with delivering treatment is that alcohol dependence is seen by government primarily as a public health issue, while drug dependence is seen essentially as a criminal justice issue—policy and funding are separate. Patients of course do not sort themselves out so conveniently.

LEAP ORIGINS AND RATIONALE

The need to increase choice and opportunity in the context of a reformulation of the national drugs policy were the driving forces to establish a National Health Service (NHS) unit to offer an alternative to maintenance treatment for those ready to move on or those who chose a different path. It was clear that cost was one potential barrier to treatment, so any model ought to be less expensive than traditional residential treatment, the modality most associated with abstinence-oriented approaches. A large recovery community in Scotland already existed with around 1,000 listed weekly mutual aid meetings nationally. The populous Central Lowlands had the greatest density of meetings, but generally, this was a resource not capitalized upon by treatment providers. William White (2007) has written of the value of recovery communities and their place in recovery maintenance, and from the outset, it was seen to be critical that such links were sought, established, and developed as the impact of treatment was likely to fade as the client moved further away from the treatment experience.

Although maintenance treatments have been extensively studied, few have looked at abstinence-oriented treatment in the United Kingdom. Some evidence does exist for the efficacy of residential rehabilitation including for cost-effectiveness. Using data from the Drug Abuse Treatment Outcome Study (DATOS), Flynn, Kristiansen, Porto, and Hubbard (1999) found a benefit from residential treatment and follow-up support in aftercare ranging from 1.7 to 2.7. NTORS and DORIS both found strong associations between residential treatment and abstinence outcomes (Gossop et al., 1997; McKeganey et al., 2004). Key elements found to be positively associated with enduring abstinence include housing, education, training and employment, psychotherapeutic interventions, therapeutic community principles and approaches (De Leon, 1984; De Leon, Jainchill, & Wexler, 1982; Lees, Manning, & Rawlings, 2004), physical and mental health care, 12-step facilitation, family support, and assertive referral to mutual aid and aftercare. In developing the Lothians and Edinburgh Abstinence Program (LEAP), the challenge was how to bring these together in an integrated way and make them work together as part of treatment delivery.

Early in the process, the aims of the service were distilled. These are:

- to offer access to quality treatment based on need and, in line with NHS principles, providing treatment free at the point of care to patients in the Lothian area;
- to help patients achieve abstinence through a biopsychosocial integrated treatment model working in partnership with other agencies;
- to increase the choice of treatment options available and to be part of a continuum of care;
- to support patients with recovery initiation and medium-term maintenance through treatment of good quality and sufficient duration;
- to help develop and build community recovery resources; and
- to demonstrate through evaluation that such a model could be effective.

Underpinning these aims were these principles:

- Patients with alcohol and drug problems should have access to the same quality of treatment as other NHS patients and be treated with the same respect.
- High aspiration: believe that people can recover from chemical dependence.

- The patient is an "expert" in the process, with staff being guides and facilitators.
- Connecting people to the recovery community locally was essential for ongoing recovery maintenance.

Meetings were held with commissioners, and it was clear that the model sat well with local priorities for "wraparound services" and integrated working. The Scottish Executive (the forerunner of the Scottish Government) was interested in funding several abstinence pilots across the country and agreed to fund the LEAP proposal as part of that. In November 2006, the funding was announced for four pilots including LEAP, and work started on finding premises, appointing a project manager, recruiting a team, and developing the program.

THE MODEL AND THE PROGRAM

The approach is that of a modified Minnesota Model but with much more focus on integrating locally available services and capitalizing on the availability of local support groups, structures, and communities. In the traditional Minnesota Model, the client is treated by a multidisciplinary team that conducts initial and ongoing assessments focused on a goal of abstinence. Interventions typically involve individual and group therapy. Elements of the 12-step philosophy underpin the model and frame addiction as an illness that needs ongoing management. These features are preserved. Where the model begins to diversify is in its direction of gaze. The LEAP model is outward facing; it looks to resources in the community, including peer support, to continue to build recovery capital both during, and most importantly, after treatment. An assumption is made that building personal recovery capital and drawing on community recovery capital are fundamental elements in the process of recovery. Furthermore, treatment can facilitate that process. LEAP is a community treatment program, embedded in the city of Edinburgh, which treats local people rather than being a regional referral center and is free to the client at the point of delivery.

The structural form is that of quasiresidential treatment. At LEAP, there are two separate sites. The multidisciplinary team is based in the day unit, which is situated within walking distance of the 16-bed supported accommodation unit. This arrangement is less expensive than a traditional residential model.

Attempting to integrate treatment with housing, education, training, and employment as well as social and recreational opportunity is a well-established principle, but its application in the United Kingdom is less well developed. There is evidence that addressing wider issues is helpful. For instance, homelessness is a risk factor for early dropout, and programs that provide housing have lower dropout rates (Dobscha, Delucchi, & Young, 1999; Tommasello, Myers, Gillis, Treherne, & Plumhoff, 1999). It was clear that accommodating people while in treatment and planning next-stage housing were likely to be helpful in determining the success of the project and to ensure good outcomes for clients. Some spaces in the program (20%) were set aside for day patients.

The value of education, training, and employment has been evidenced (Joe, Chastain, Marsh, & Simpson, 1985; Simpson & Marsh, 1986), and it was planned from the outset that such an initiative should be integrated into the LEAP program. Group work as part of therapy has advantages, and this may act through support, affiliation, and identification mechanisms (Leshner, 1997; Project Match Research Group, 1997). There is evidence of the benefit of combining treatment and 12-step approaches—identified by Humphreys (2004)—and this was adopted. National Institute of Clinical Excellence (2007) guidelines recommend that families and carers be involved in assessment and treatment (p. 72), that mutual aid be offered to clients (p. 55), and that psychological interventions be employed (p. 116), so these were integrated into the model.

Based on existing evidence and guidelines, the key components of the service were planned to be:

- Medical: an assessment of mental and physical health with a care plan developed to attend to any unmet needs. Detoxification is offered.
- Therapeutic: three levels of therapeutic intervention involving group psychotherapy, one-to-one counseling, and the effect of the therapeutic community. The model would be eclectic and use motivational interviewing techniques, person-centered approaches, and cognitive behavioral elements.
- Housing: attending to housing needs both while in treatment and after treatment. Other social needs would need to be identified and addressed and would include financial and criminal justice issues.
- Access to education, training, and employment.
- Assertive linkage to mutual aid and recovery communities.
- Provision of aftercare in the longer term.
- The provision of structured and meaningful activities.
- Addressing exercise and nutrition.

Patients have both medical and therapeutic care plans, which are developed in partnership between patients and staff. Recreation, exercise, and alternative therapies are included. The therapeutic community has a hierarchy with senior peers, a group leader, and a deputy. Various duties are shared by members of the community. Reviews involving key individuals are held at midpoint (6 weeks) and prior to discharge. A graduation ceremony celebrates the success of individuals in completing the program as they move on to take up aftercare support.

ESTABLISHING THE SERVICE: PROGRESS AND CHALLENGES

Establishing partnerships was an early priority. From the outset, managers from the housing department in the City of Edinburgh Council saw the value in the proposal and were keen to seek solutions. They agreed to dedicate one of the city's homeless hostels to the project for 2 years. A voluntary sector (nongovernment organization) partner (Transition/Access to Industry) was engaged to deliver a session a week to our patients who were preparing for education, training, and employment and to provide more intensive services after program completion.

A meeting was held in Edinburgh to which representatives of the mutual aid groups were invited, and while their traditions discouraged affiliation, a spirit of cooperation was evident with the meeting well attended and the project gaining support. An official launch half-day was also held, and representatives of potential referring agencies were invited, with around 100 people attending.

The duration of the funding was just over 2 years, which meant challenges existed in terms of proving and evaluating the project. Recruiting an experienced staff team was a priority as there was little time to train staff unfamiliar with a recovery model. Many of the therapy staff had experience working in residential settings, and all had significant experience in group facilitation.

As funders, the government in Scotland took a keen interest in the development of the project and hosted regular support meetings for representatives of all the pilots. The government provided guidance through the evaluation-tendering process and encouraged the collection of data on throughputs, quality, and outcomes.

In view of the polarization of the harm reduction/abstinence debate in the United Kingdom, it was important to place the new service firmly within a range of options that NHS Lothian offered through the Substance Misuse Directorate. However, from the outset, it was clear that there was work to be done to address expressed concerns and to generate confidence in the service. Doubts were expressed about the feasibility of trying to detoxify and treat substance-dependent patients in a community environment, the received wisdom from residential treatment providers being that such cases needed isolation to recover. Many of the concerns that were raised were similar to those addressed in the Recovery Academy's "Straw Men" article (Best et al., 2010).

Concerns were raised that we were potentially setting people up to fail and that the danger inherent in abstinence (loss of tolerance, risk for relapse, overdose, and death) was too high. We were able to allay some of these concerns by explaining what steps we were taking to introduce harm reduction education and by addressing loss of tolerance and prevention of overdose. On assessment, admission, and discharge and at intervals during treatment, education is given on reducing the risk. If relapse is to happen, we advise service users not to inject, not to use alone, not to mix drugs, and to use less of the substance than before. Written material is also provided.

Another concern was around the 12-step components of the program. With evidence that many UK treatment professionals hold ambivalent or negative views (Day, Gaston, Furlong, Murali, & Copello, 2005), this was not a surprise. Patients referred to LEAP, however, demonstrated that this was not a concern of theirs (Figure 8, 2008, p. 37). From the outset, there were concerns that the model did not suit the needs of single parents with children. Among residential (Tier 4) services, this is an acknowledged problem; there are few units in the United Kingdom able to accommodate parents and children. LEAP has attempted to create flexible programs for parents with childcare responsibilities.

GROUPS AT LEAP

Groups feature at LEAP in various guises and with several functions. Daily-facilitated groups (two groups of 10 service users) allow peer-to-peer support, encounter, and challenge to happen. The practice of interpersonal skills and experience of the group process help to catalyze the social and psychological change required to build recovery capital. Groups last an hour. Other groups include relapse prevention, personal effectiveness training, men's and women's groups, goal-setting group, an early intervention group for lapse and relapse, and three aftercare groups per week. Weekend planning meetings with the entire peer group present allow preparation for that part of the week that many with substance misuse problems find challenging. On a Monday, weekend process takes place where peers analyze difficult moments and celebrate the successes of the weekend. On a Thursday, the entire community, peer supporters, and staff team meet to take stock of the health of the therapeutic community and to highlight any concerns about behavior or vulnerability of peers. Groups also exist in the community, and assertive referral is made to these. They include mutual aid groups, service user groups, and peer-led and recreational groups.

EVALUATING PROCESS AND OUTCOMES

Following a tendering process, the external evaluation of LEAP was conducted by Figure 8 Consultancy Limited. Internal monitoring has also been conducted. The quality of the service was found to be good and much more advanced than might be expected for a new initiative. Detailed outcomes will be published in due course and are deliberately not the focus of this article; however, some key findings are outlined here.

The mean age of LEAP patients is 34 years old. Patients have a higher-than-average Severity of Dependence Score of 12.7 versus a score of 11.1 as reported in the national outcome study DORIS (Figure 8, 2010a). Forty-three percent of service users are homeless on admission. The service has had almost 900 referrals in 3 years of operation. In 2009 to 2010, there were 327 referrals and 113 admissions, with men accounting for 70% of these. The predominant referrers are the specialist drug services, general practitioners, and housing agencies. Six out of 10 patients admitted to the service are detoxified in the community while on the program. Detoxification is offered from alcohol, opiates, and benzodiazepines using locally developed detoxification regimes.

An internally conducted follow-up of the first 103 graduates found that 60% remained alcohol and drug free, with durations of continuous recovery ranging from 3 months to nearly 2 years. In the formal outcome study, the graduate groups reported significant positive changes in satisfaction with work, alcohol use, drug use, legal situation, and family and other relationships. The evaluation reported a retention (completion) rate of 64%, with service users reporting high levels of satisfaction across a range of measures using the Treatment Perception Questionnaire (Figure 8, 2008, p. 43). The following are illustrative quotes from service users from the evaluation:

> Being an alcoholic and being in psychiatric hospitals three times, I have never had the back-up before this and so relapsed. LEAP offered me ongoing care and aftercare for the next 2 years which I will find very beneficial for my ongoing treatment. (Figure 8, 2008, p. 15)

> I am able to handle situations I couldn't before. LEAP is helping me to achieve goals—family problems are sorted and [I have] training opportunities for future. (Figure 8, 2008, p. 23)

> Found out going to group meetings [Alcoholics Anonymous (AA), Narcotics Anonymous (NA), and Cocaine Anonymous (CA)], which I strongly disapproved of before treatment, have actually been richly rewarding—building up self-esteem, respect etc. Mainly by listening and sharing—talking in public or in a group was never my strong point and can still improve more." (Figure 8, 2008, p. 48)

Improvements in abstinence rates were found across all substances in graduates from the program at 9-month follow up, and injecting reduced from an average of 4.5 days in the previous 30 days to 0 days.

The evaluators suggested a savings-to-cost ratio of the service of 3 to 1 and highly rated the quality of the service. A LEAP peer supporter and a volunteer were recently honored with awards for their roles in the project, and the LEAP partners won an award for partnership working in 2010.

The early outcomes (9 months) identified in the LEAP evaluation (Figure 8, 2010a) will be built on by results from a longer-term follow up with a cohort of 144 individuals, and this will be published in due course.

LEADING THE WAY

In the spirit of encouraging those in recovery through treatment to make a difference in policy and practice, we have encouraged our graduates to take up opportunities where they arise. The hope is that this will open up more pathways to recovery for others and also will build recovery capital in those involved and in the community. A significant support early in the life of LEAP was the reference to the program in the body of the government's national drug strategy document as an example of good practice (Scottish Government, 2008, p. 25). The Drugs Policy Unit consulted our patients prior to, during, and after the launch of the policy document. LEAP graduates endure recovery work in a volunteering role on various national bodies, including the National Forum on Drug-Related Deaths in Scotland, the Drugs Strategy Delivery Commission, the Scottish Drugs Forum, and the Scottish Drugs Recovery Consortium, and sit on various local committees in Lothian.

In 2009, NHS Lothian opened up work placement opportunities for LEAP graduates in a variety of settings within the health service locally. This offers a practical opportunity to gain employment experience, and it is hoped that a significant number of these will convert into employment posts. The service has seen many visitors in its short life, with more than 500 people in total attending the monthly open days. LEAP has also hosted members of parliament, members of the Scottish Parliament, UK Government ministers, and Scottish Government ministers. There have been visits from delegations or individuals from the United States, Canada, Denmark, Norway, and Greece, not to mention Alcohol and Drug Partnership (ADP) and drug service visits from many parts of Scotland and England. The reason for many visits has been to understand what is happening and to explore whether it is transferable.

As patients have maintained their recoveries after graduation and continued to take advantage of the aftercare program, there has been growing interest in peers contributing to the support of the patients currently in the treatment program. This is encouraged, and the entire staff team was trained in supervision techniques to provide regular support. Peer supporters act as role models to current patients, support the therapeutic community and individuals in it, and accompany patients to appointments at hospital, the Benefits Agency, the local general practitioner, to legal appointments, etc. They also take part in weekend activities. As it grows, peer support will be developed in a more structured way, with consideration given to training, role definition, and boundaries as well as to offering training in recovery coaching. Other agencies are now looking at introducing peer support, and LEAP will pass on experience and learning wherever it is asked.

BRIDGING THE GAP: RELATIONSHIPS WITH LOCAL COMMUNITIES OF RECOVERY

Recognition of the value of recovery communities has been an important principle at LEAP from the outset. Mark Litt and colleagues from the University of Connecticut have shown that increasing the number of sober people in one's social network is associated with higher abstinence rates for those with alcohol problems (Litt, Kadden, Kabela-Cormier, & Petry, 2009). Building bridges to those sober communities and helping to nurture and consolidate them has been vital. The most tangible face of this community locally is represented in the existing mutual aid fellowship groups. In 2006, the year before LEAP began treating patients, according to their respective Web sites, there were 10 mutual aid groups operating in Lothian aimed at supporting abstinence in drug misusers. Today there are 23 meetings of NA and CA listed in the area. LEAP's relationship to this growth is of interest, and while it is not possible to prove causality, it is noteworthy that many of the key volunteer service positions in the area structures of these groups and in the individual groups themselves are graduates of LEAP (LEAP Service User Group, personal communication, July 2010). In addition to NA and CA, AA has a strong local presence, with around 90 weekly meetings in Lothian. A Self-Management and Recovery Training (SMART) Recovery group, offering mutual aid based on cognitive behavioral principles, has just launched in Lothian and is a welcome addition to the resources on offer.

The linkage of patients to local recovery communities and evidencing the reality of recovery is enhanced by having aftercare sessions three times weekly at our base. A large group of graduates attending regularly attest to current patients that recovery is a reality and that there are many people "making it" out there. We encourage the groups to mix. We also invite past peers to come back to share their stories with current patients, which is mutually beneficial.

More recently, LEAP has been operating in collaboration with the Serenity Café. A social enterprise, the café holds monthly themed nights offering a safe social space for recovering people to gather and celebrate recovery connecting to others as they do so. Many of the volunteers at the Serenity Café are LEAP graduates as are many of the customers. The Serenity Café has recently won a "community action" award for community development. An additional award for volunteering was also achieved.

The Serenity Café has also developed a football (soccer) team, on which LEAP graduates play, and more recently a women's group, which our clients will also benefit from. Although LEAP is well represented here, another advantage of partnership and engagement with the Serenity Café is exposure of our graduates to others who have been through different treatment types and who have different experiences of recovery. On café nights, patients in the program are encouraged to go along to enjoy themselves and experience that this is possible without having to use alcohol or drugs. Further developments already include a recovery drama group, and there are plans to have a recovery choir in the city.

The newly dubbed "LEAP Partnership" of LEAP, the City of Edinburgh Council, Access to Industry (Transition), and the Serenity Café is exploring how we can work more closely together and help and support recovering people to develop communities of recovery locally. An example is the planning and facilitation of a Lothian recovery-community corporate presence at the 2010 National Recovery Walk in Glasgow. All members of the partnership are clear that supporting the development of a strong and inclusive recovery community locally is the key to sustained recovery not just for those completing treatment but for many of those recovering in other ways.

Other less formal recovery initiatives developing locally include recovery football (soccer), the LEAP guitar club, a recovery arts group, a recent recovery rock concert attracting hundreds of people, and even a recovery chess league. It is difficult to gauge the extent of the wider informal supportive social networks supporting recovering people as they meet in cafés and homes or share in recreational activities.

A recovery community needs to be embedded in wider communities, and LEAP staff meets annually with neighbors and with the local council of churches in the neighborhood of our treatment center. Local faith communities and individuals from these communities have supported our patients financially. The part these wider, mostly posttreatment interventions and supports play is likely to be considerable in helping clients sustain recovery.

DISCUSSION AND KEY LESSONS

It has been demonstrated that delivering a recovery treatment and rehabilitation program in a community setting from within the health service with partners is feasible. Establishing close links with the recovery community has been achieved and is still developing. The value of meaningful activity through structured opportunities into education, employment, and aftercare has been reported by patients. The celebration of recovery is becoming more prominent locally and is evidenced through "sell out" graduation ceremonies, volunteering and other awards, press coverage, and growth in size of mutual aid groups.

After 3 years of operation, we are able to point to some of the strengths of the service. Looking outward, valuing recovery communities as the power-house of recovery maintenance and catalyzing the development of peer sup-port have been cornerstones in the work we do. Our current and ex-patients, however, are the experts here, and capitalizing on their lived experience of recovery has undoubtedly yielded results in terms of retention in treatment and in outcomes. There is a satisfying loop of support going on as those learning how to maintain recovery pass on their knowledge to their own benefit and the benefit of others. This "collective recovery capital" seems to be an important factor in sustaining recovery and merits further study.

Other strengths of the service include the practice of assertive linkage to the recovery community, having high aspirations for service users, and delivering a positive treatment experience. It is difficult to capture important intangibles such as staff enthusiasm and energy, the welcoming environment and atmosphere, and the presence of hope, which many who visit comment on, yet they are all there and part of success.

As understanding grows over the important but limited role for treatment and of the great need to develop effective systems for ongoing care and encourage the growth of the recovery community, more energy has gone into supporting this at LEAP. We have learned that while treatment is an important "step up" into recovery for some, sustaining these gains has much more to do with strong recovery communities.

In the recently published needs assessment for drug and alcohol prob-lems in the city of Edinburgh, two of the seven recommendations were specific to recovery communities (Figure 8, 2010b, p. 2). These were:

- The planning and development of services to meet these needs should be built around the ambitions of service users and their families within a recovery-orientated system of care. Developing services in this way will provide benefits to people who use the service but will also help de-velop community-based mutual aid and peer support networks, thereby enhancing the ability for people to move on from services.
- In terms of prioritization of needs, it is recommended that any further reinvestment of resources should initially be targeted at enhancing the posttreatment phase of recovery, while supporting and developing recov-ery communities across the city.

The value of forming bonds with other recovery-oriented treatment ser-vices and initiatives both locally and nationally has become a learning point for LEAP. We are perhaps better placed now to help colleagues in other services understand the potential benefits of assertive referral to mutual aid. In the City of Edinburgh Needs Assessment (Figure 8, 2010b), only 0.4% of those service users surveyed ($n = 249$) were attending a drug-specific mutual aid group; 0.8% of the sample was attending AA. These are low up-take rates by any standard and raise questions about why these resources are not being utilized.

At LEAP, the team saw the development of the Serenity Café as a significant boost to the local recovery community. We have learned how to work in collaborative partnership for the benefit of clients. Despite being connected by the 12-step program, there is still a lack of overlap and traffic between NA, CA, and AA locally. The Serenity Café allows for divisions to come down and for shared experience to bring people together. In addition, those whose recovery has not involved mutual aid groups also attend café nights, which increases the spectrum of different types of recovery journeys represented in a broader community.

In the current difficult fiscal setting, it may be challenging to further develop the LEAP model in terms of a rollout or even locally, although there are good reasons to look at doing precisely this. Gathering further information on longer-term outcomes from the LEAP community treatment program will help determine if short-term gains can be sustained. Trying to make the model more flexible to meet the needs of more clients is a goal for the future. The service does not currently serve the needs of those with childcare responsibilities as well as we would like, and this is another area where recovery community resources may be developed and brought to bear.

THE FUTURE

NHS Lothian has commissioned a longer-term follow-up that will track patients' outcomes, but we also need to develop other methods of mapping growth and development of the recovery community, peer support, and transfer of individual recovery experience. Further developing the service in ways that continue to draw on the resources of the recovery community is a priority for LEAP. We need to find ways of passing on the lessons learned to policymakers, commissioners, other services, and colleagues. Celebrating the success of those who have recovered from dependent drug and alcohol use will in turn allow others to experience the same success by showcasing the reality of recovery. It is hoped that recovery communities locally will reach a tipping point where growth in peer-supported services, mutual aid groups, and other community recovery resources will become self-sustaining, and treatment will be seen as an adjunct to mutual aid and peer-based recovery support rather than the other way round.

REFERENCES

Best, D., Bamber, S., Battersby, A., Gilman, M., Groshkova, T., Honor, S., ... White, W. (2010). Recovery and straw men: An analysis of the objections raised to the transition to a recovery model in UK addiction services. *Journal of Groups in Addiction and Recovery, 5*(3), 264–288.

Best, D., Groshkova, T., & McTague, P. (2009, July/August). The politics of numbers. *Druglink*, 14–17.

Best, D., O'Grady, A., Charalampous, I., & Gordon, D. (2005). *National needs assessment of tier 4 drug treatment services in England*. London, UK: National Treatment Agency.

Day, E., Gaston, R. L., Furlong, E., Murali, V., & Copello, A. (2005). United Kingdom substance misuse treatment workers' attitudes toward 12-step self-help groups. *Journal of Substance Abuse Treatment, 29*(4), 321–327.

De Leon, G. (1984). *The therapeutic community: Study of effectiveness* (National Institute on Drug Abuse Research Monograph Series [DHHS Publication No. ADM:84-1286]). Rockville, MD: National Institute on Drug Abuse.

De Leon, G., Jainchill, N., & Wexler, H. (1982). Success and improvement rates 5 years after treatment in a therapeutic community. *International Journal of Addictions, 17*(4), 703–747.

Dobscha, S., Delucchi, K., & Young, M. (1999). Adherence with referrals for outpatient follow-up from a VA psychiatry emergency room. *Community Mental Health Journal, 35*, 451–458.

Figure 8. (2008). *LEAP at 1 year: Evaluation of Lothian and Edinburgh Abstinence Program*. Dundee, UK: Figure 8 Consultancy Services.

Figure 8. (2010a). *Lothians and Edinburgh Abstinence Program: Final evaluation report*. Dundee: Figure 8 Consultancy Services.

Figure 8. (2010b). *Needs assessment of drug and alcohol problems in Edinburgh city: Report prepared for Edinburgh Alcohol and Drugs Partnership*. Dundee: Figure 8 Consultancy Services.

Flynn, P. M. Kristiansen, P. L., Porto, J. V., & Hubbard, R. L. (1999). Cost and benefits of cocaine addiction in DATOS. *Drug and Alcohol Dependence, 57*(2), 167–174.

Gossop, M., Marsden, J., Stewart, D., Edwards, C., Lehmann, P., Wilson, A., & Segar, G. (1997). The National Treatment Research Outcome Study in the United Kingdom: Six-month follow-up outcomes. *Psychology of Addictive Behaviors, 11*, 324–337.

Griesbach, D., Russell, P., Duff, L., O'Brien, K., Rich, C., & Thompson, S. (2004). *Residential detoxification and rehabilitation services for drug users: A review*. Edinburgh, Scotland: Effective Interventions Unit, Scottish Executive, Edinburgh.

Hay, G., Gannon, M., Casey, J., & McKeganey, N. (2009). *Estimating the local and national prevalence of problem drug use in Scotland*. Edinburgh, Scotland: ISD Scotland.

Humphreys, K. (2004). *Circles of recovery: Self-help organizations for addictions*. Cambridge, UK: Cambridge University Press.

Joe, G. W., Chastain, R. L., Marsh, K. L., & Simpson, D. D. (1985). *Opioid recidivism factors: 12-year follow-up of 1969–72 admissions to DARP drug abuse treatments*. College Station, TX: Texas A&M University, Behavioral Research Program.

Lees, J., Manning, N., & Rawlings, B. (2004). A culture of enquiry: Research evidence and the therapeutic community. *Psychiatric Quarterly, 75*, 279–294.

Leshner, A. I. (1997). Introduction to the special issue: The National Institute on Drug Abuse's Drug Treatment Outcome Study (DATOS). *Psychology of Addictive Behaviors, 11*(4), 211–215.

Litt, M. D., Kadden, R. M., Kabela-Cormier, E., & Petry, N. M. (2009). Changing network support for drinking: Network support project 2-year follow up. *Journal of Consulting and Clinical Psychology, 77*(2), 229–242.

McKeganey, N., Bloor, M., Robertson, M., Neale, J., & MacDougall, J. (2006). Abstinence and drug abuse treatment: Results from the Drug Outcome Research in Scotland Study. *Drugs: Education, Prevention, and Policy, 13*(6), 537–550.

McKeganey, N., Morris, Z., Neale, J., & Robertson, M. (2004). What are drug users looking for when they contact drug services: Abstinence or harm reduction? *Drugs: Education Prevention and Policy, 11*(5), 423–435.

National Treatment Agency. (2002). *Models of Care for the treatment of drug misusers: Promoting quality, efficiency, and effectiveness in drug treatment services in England.* London, UK: Author.

National Institute of Clinical Excellence. (2007). *Drug misuse: Psychosocial interventions* (National Clinical Practice Guideline Number 51). London, UK: National Institute for Clinical Excellence.

Project Match Research Group. (1997). Matching alcoholism treatments to client heterogeneity: Project Match posttreatment drinking outcomes. *Journal of Studies on Alcohol, 58*(1), 7–29.

Scottish Advisory Committee on Drug Misuse. (2008). *Essential care: A report on the approach required to maximize opportunity for recovery from problem substance use in Scotland.* Edinburgh, Scotland: Author.

Scottish Advisory Committee on Drug Misuse Methadone Project Group. (2007). *Reducing harm and promoting recovery: A report on methadone treatment for substance misuse in Scotland.* Edinburgh, Scotland: Scottish Advisory Council on Drug Misuse.

Scottish Government. (2007). *Review of methadone in drug treatment: Prescribing information and practice.* Retrieved from http://www.scotland.gov.uk/Resource/Doc/180406/0051268.pdf

Scottish Government. (2008). *The road to recovery: A new approach to tackling Scotland's drug problem.* Edinburgh, Scotland: Author.

Simpson, D. D., & Marsh, K. L. (1986). *Relapse and recovery among opioid addicts 12 years after treatment.* College Station, TX: Texas A&M University, Behavioral Research Program.

Tommasello, A. C., Myers, C. P., Gillis, L., Treherne, L. L., & Plumhoff, M. (1999). Effectiveness of outreach to homeless substance abusers. *Evaluation and Program Planning, 22,* 296–303.

White, W. (2007). Addiction recovery: Its definition and conceptual boundaries. *Journal of Substance Abuse Treatment, 33,* 229–241.

Recovery Group Participation Scale (RGPS): Factor Structure in Alcohol and Heroin Recovery Populations

TEODORA GROSHKOVA

National Addiction Center, Institute of Psychiatry, King's College London, London, United Kingdom

DAVID BEST

Center for Criminal Justice and Policing, University of the West of Scotland, Hamilton, Lanarkshire, Scotland, United Kingdom

WILLIAM WHITE

Addiction Studies, Chestnut Health Systems, Punta Gorda, Florida, USA

Recovery group participation is relevant to both clinical and research activity. Its measurement with the Recovery Group Participation Scale (RGPS) is an attempt to have a measurement of participation across a range of recovery groups. The factor structure, among other psychometric properties of the scale, is however, undefined. The present study examined the factor structure of the RGPS in alcohol and drug recovery populations in Birmingham and Glasgow, United Kingdom. Participants from the Birmingham (n = 219) and Glasgow (n = 205) recovery studies who had a completed form of the RGPS formed the basis for the factor structure examination. Principal component analysis extracted one factor, which accounted for 39.3% and 67.4% in the Birmingham and the Glasgow samples, respectively. Overall scores on the RGPS were associated with higher quality-of-life scores and with greater self-esteem and social networks of nonusers in recovery. The key question that remains to be addressed is the evolving role of recovery group participation in prospective studies of growth of recovery capital and sustained recovery.

INTRODUCTION

Addiction recovery mutual aid groups have a long history (White, 1998, 2004) and in recent decades have experienced dramatic growth, extensive specialization (by drug choice and membership characteristics, e.g., special meetings for women, young people, and people with co-occurring disorders), philosophical diversification (explicitly religious, spiritual, and secular frameworks of recovery; moderation-based groups), wide geographical dispersion, and new delivery platforms (e.g., Internet-based recovery communities; Humphreys, 2004; White, 2004; White & Kurtz, 2006). Orienting individuals to the benefits of recovery mutual aid groups, particularly Alcoholics Anonymous (AA) and other 12-step groups, and linking clients to these groups have become mainstream practices in many addiction treatment programs, particularly in the United States (Roman & Blum, 1997).

Research evaluating the effects of participation in recovery mutual aid societies has increased in tandem with these trends, as have the controversies surrounding the interpretation of the major study findings (Kaskutas, 2009). These controversies stem in part from the weak methodological rigor of early studies (Humphreys, 2006). Improved measurement, longer follow-up periods, higher follow-up rates, and the use of comparison groups have elevated the quality of more recent studies (Kelly & Yeterian, 2008), but a persistent and pervasive limitation is the near-exclusive focus of these studies on AA and to a lesser extent adaptations of AA's 12-step program (e.g., Narcotics Anonymous [NA] and Cocaine Anonymous). Only a few (mostly descriptive) studies have been conducted on such secular recovery support groups as LifeRing Secular Recovery (White & Nicolaus, 2005), Secular Organization for Sobriety (Connors & Dermen, 1996), Women for Sobriety, Smart Recovery (Horvath, 1999/2000), and Moderation Management (Humphreys, 2003; Humphreys & Klaw, 2001). Particularly noteworthy by their absence are scientific studies of explicitly religious addiction recovery support groups (e.g., Alcoholics Victorious, Alcoholics for Christ, Calix Society, Celebrate Recovery, Jewish Alcoholics, Chemically Dependent People and Significant Others, and Millati Islami; White, 2009). AA's dominance as a focus of research is understandable in light of its membership size, worldwide dispersion, and its frequent adaptation to other addictions and problems of living, but it is unclear the extent to which findings of AA studies can be extended to other addiction recovery mutual aid groups (White, 2009).

Studies of AA have focused primarily on such issues as the: (1) overall effectiveness of AA (including three meta-analyses; Emrick, Tonigan, Montgomery, & Little, 1993; Kownacki & Shadish, 1999; Tonigan, Toscova, & Miller, 1996); (2) potent ingredients of AA (Moos, 2008; Morgenstern,

Labouvie, McCray, Kahler, & Frey, 1997); (3) response variability to AA across individuals and demographic and clinical subpopulations (e.g., women, adolescents, people of color, people with co-occurring psychiatric disorders, and people low in religiosity; Hillhouse & Fiorentine, 2001; Kelly, Myers, & Brown, 2002; Morgenstern, Kahler, Frey, & Labouvie, 1996); (4) dose and duration effects of AA participation (Humphreys, Moos, & Cohen, 1997; Kaskutas et al., 2005); (5) the effects of timing (pretreatment, in treatment, posttreatment) of linkage and linkage procedures to AA (Kaskutas, Subbaraman, Witbrodt, & Zemore, 2009; Moos & Moos, 2004); and (6) the cost-effectiveness of recovery mutual aid participation (Humphreys & Moos, 1996, 2001).

There is growing scientific consensus that participation in a recovery mutual aid group can exert significant effects on the long-term resolution of alcohol and other drug problems (for reviews, see Humphreys, 2004; Humphreys et al., 2004; Kelly & Yeterian, 2008; White, 2009). Efforts to isolate the active ingredients of recovery mutual aid involvement have focused on several factors, including problem recognition and commitment to change, regular remotivation, social network reconstruction, spirituality, enhanced coping skills, and therapeutic effects of helping others (Bond, Kaskutas, & Weisner, 2003; Kelly et al., 2000; Laudet, Cleland, Magura, Vogel, & Knight, 2004; Longabaugh, Wirtz, Zweben, & Stout, 1998; Morgenstern et al., 1997; Zemore, Kaskutas, & Ammon, 2004). The larger finding that intensity of mutual aid participation is a critical factor in predicting recovery outcomes may be linked to the activation and amplification of multiple potent ingredients (Cacciola, Dugosh, Foltz, Leahy, & Stevens, 2005; Humphreys, Moos, & Cohen, 1997; Montgomery, Miller, & Tonigan, 1995; Sheeren, 1988; Toumbourou, Hamilton, U'Ren, Stevens-Jones, & Storey, 2002).

Several instruments have been developed to measure AA affiliation and intensity of participation. Earlier instruments, such as the "Steps Questionnaire" (Gilbert, 1991), have focused exclusively on AA-related beliefs, missing out the opportunity to tap other aspects of participation in AA, such as meeting attendance activity. Adaptive evolution in the field has resulted in the development and validation of the recovery interview (Morgenstern et al., 1996), the widely used AA Involvement Scale (Tonigan, Connors, & Miller, 1996), and the AA Affiliation Scale (Humphreys, Kaskutas, & Weisner, 1998). More recently, instruments such as the Global Appraisal of Individual Needs (Dennis, Titus, White, Unsicker, & Hodgkins, 2002) have been developed; these include subscales that measure intensity of AA/NA participation. Most such scales combine items measuring group attendance with those assessing participation in specific nonmeeting activities. However, the use of many of these instruments and subscales is limited when applied to the growing menu of non-12-step recovery mutual aid groups. An additional concern regarding these measures is that they have been created using data from U.S. research. So, the norms for these instruments may not generalize to a UK setting.

The purpose of the present study is to test a Recovery Group Participation Scale (RGPS) that could measure intensity of participation in all recovery support groups. This scale, developed initially as a tool to be used by probation officers to measure recovery mutual aid involvement of probationers (White & Gasperin, 2006), has been used in the United States and the United Kingdom, but no studies have been conducted on its factorial structure. The authors examine the factor structure of the scale, based on two UK samples of individuals in recovery from dependence on alcohol or heroin.

METHODS

Study Participants and Procedures

The sample consisted of 424 alcohol- and drug-recovering addicts, who were participating in two studies of recovery journeys in Birmingham, England ($n = 219$), and Glasgow, Scotland ($n = 205$). The methods and main questions of the two parent recovery studies have been described elsewhere (Best, Gow, et al., in press; Best, Groshkova, et al., in press). In brief, based on a peer snowballing method, the study in Birmingham recruited 24 members of DATUS, a service users' group for both abstinent and maintained clients in contact with drug treatment services in Birmingham. These individuals were then trained to deliver a structured research instrument and asked to identify and interview members of their peer networks who fulfilled the study inclusion criteria and who were willing to participate in the study. Each volunteer was asked to recruit individuals who (1) reported lifetime heroin dependence, (2) had been abstinent from heroin in the last year, and (3) perceived themselves as "recovered" or "in recovery." This resulted in a sample of 219. The study in Glasgow had built on the methods used in Birmingham and supplemented snowballing with recruitment through recovery groups (including 12-step and other mutual aid organizations such as SMART recovery and "nontherapeutic" recovery groups) and advertisement in the local press, targeting not only former heroin users but extending the project to include individuals and groups relating to recovery from other substances including alcohol. Thus, 107 problem drinkers and 98 former heroin users, both in long-term maintenance treatment ($n = 37$) and nonmaintained and abstinent from illicit drugs ($n = 61$), took part in this study.

Measures

At both localities, the interview schedule consisted of measures including validated indicators of psychological and physical health and quality of life; self-esteem and self-efficacy; lifetime and last month drug use; and severity of dependence (Table 1).

TABLE 1 Instruments Used to Assess Functioning

Measure (Acronym)	Description and domains measured	Scoring	Source of psychometrics
Assessment of Recovery Capital (ARC)	A 100-item measure assessing recovery strengths and threats to recovery in 10 domains.	Range of scores for each scale is 0 to 5 (recovery strengths) and 0 to 5 (threats to recovery)	Best & Groshkova (2011)
The World Health Organization Quality of Life-BREF (WHOQOL-BREF)	A shorter (26-item) version of the original instrument (World Health Organization, 1993), measuring the broad domains of physical and psychological health, social relationships, and environmental quality of life.	Raw scores are transformed to a score between 0 and 100. Higher scores signify higher functioning.	WHOQOL Group (1998a, 1998b)
Client Evaluation of Self and Treatment (CEST): Self-efficacy and self-esteem	Accepted research and clinical measure assessing client needs and performance in the areas of: treatment motivation (desire for help, treatment readiness, needs, and pressures), psychological functioning (self-esteem, depression, anxiety, decision-making, self-efficacy), social functioning (hostility, risk taking, social consciousness), therapeutic engagement (treatment satisfaction, rapport, treatment participation), and social network support (peer support, social support).	Scores for each subscale are averaged and multiplied by 10 to give a score between 10 and 50. Higher scores signify higher functioning	Joe, Broome, Rowan-Szal, & Simpson (2002)
The Lifetime Drug Use History (LDUH)	Research and clinical instrument available for recording the longitudinal course of a drug-using "career" using a monthly mapping of drug use patterns in relation to other life events.	n/a	Best et al. (2008) Day et al. (2008)

In addition, as part of the structured interview section, the 18-item version of the RGPS was completed by each participant in the two recovery studies. The original version of the scale consisted of 27 items and this was edited down, to allow consistency in scoring, to an 18-item, and finally, in the present study, to a 15-item self-completion questionnaire (enclosed in the Appendix); each scored between 0 and 3—giving a total score of 0 to 45.

Statistics

Factor analysis was performed on the 18-item RGPS. The criterion chosen to determine that an extracted factor accounted for a reasonably large proportion of the total variance was based on an eigenvalue greater than 1. A principal component analysis (PCA) procedure was chosen because this method is particularly useful in exploring the data while reducing multidimensionality (Jolliffe, 2002). Because there was a possibility that the principal components (factors) extracted may be correlated, a nonorthogonal factor rotation procedure was chosen (West, 1991). The determination of an appropriate item factor loading level is variable across studies (Munro, 2001) and generally ranges from 0.30 to 0.55. Kline (2000) has stipulated that a factor loading of 0.30 or greater is a salient and capable level for defining a factor. The determination of a significant item factor loading was based on Kline's criteria and set at a coefficient level of 0.40 or greater; this level was also based on a rationale of maximizing the possible number of items loading on emerging factors to generate a more complete interpretation of the data set.

The number of participants required for a factor analysis to be conducted is arbitrarily defined, with recommendations based either on absolute minimum participant numbers (Kline, 2000; Nunnally & Bernstein, 1994) or a ratio of participants to variables (Barrett & Kline, 1981; West, 1991). Under the absolute minimum participant numbers approach, a minimum of 100 participants is suggested (Kline, 2000). In contrast, the ratio-of-participants-to-variables approach stipulates a minimum ratio of three participants to each variable (West, 1991), though even ratios as low as 2 to 1 have been demonstrated to produce robust and clearly defined factors (Barrett & Kline, 1981). The approach taken in the current study is consistent with both approaches. PCA was performed on the Birmingham ($n = 219$) and Glasgow ($n = 205$) cohort data to satisfy the minimum-participant-numbers approach. However, the ratio-of-participants-to-variables approach does provide a statistically robust context to perform a PCA on each Glasgow subgroup to investigate the possible impact of primary substance abuse on the RGPS factor structure. Using the ratio of three participants to one variable, the number of participants in each group exceeds this minimum and therefore allows the analysis to be performed at the level of each subgroup. It is important to note that as an exploratory technique, PCA is not an exact statistical science, there are a number of statistical approaches that can be taken within a factor analysis, and many of these are operationally defined by arbitrarily defined minima (Kline).

Ethics

Ethical approval for the study was obtained from the local research Ethics Committees of Birmingham University and the University of the West of Scotland for the Birmingham and Glasgow samples, respectively. Written informed consent was obtained from all participants prior to the commencement of the study.

RESULTS

The two studies recruited a total of 424 alcohol- and drug-recovering addicts. One hundred individuals (mean age $= 32.8\pm7.6$ years) were recruited to the study in Birmingham and defined themselves as being in recovery from heroin use for at least 1 year (the mean reported time since last heroin use was 3.9 years). The majority of the sample was male (76%), of White British background (71%), and single (73%). More than a quarter of them reported to have been engaged in some form of meaningful activity (full- and part-time work, as well as engagement in studies or volunteering work) in the month preceding the interview (Best, Groshkova, et al., in press). In Glasgow, both former drinkers ($n = 107$) and former heroin users ($n = 98$) were recruited, and the two groups shared a similar demographic profile—mostly male (61% and 74% in the two samples, respectively), describing themselves as White British (95% and nearly 100%), and single (59% and 77%; Best, Gow, et al., in press). Among those who were recovering from alcohol, 79% reported at least some meaningful activity in the last month, while in the heroin subcohort the proportion was 53%.

Stage 1: 18-Item Version

How much variance does each factor account for? After performing a PCA, the initial eigenvalues were converted into a percentage of variance accounted for by dividing them by their sum. As shown in Table 2, 66% of the variation can be accounted for by the first five linear components (factors; the variances have been scaled to add up to 18, the number of variables or factors).

TABLE 2 Initial Eigenvalues From PCA Fit

Factor	Variance	Variance %	Cumulative %
1	6.169	34.270	34.270
2	2.105	11.694	45.965
3	1.505	8.361	54.326
4	1.085	6.028	60.353
5	1.031	5.729	66.082
6	0.897	4.985	71.067
7	0.836	4.645	75.711
8	0.750	4.165	79.876
9	0.581	3.226	83.102
10	0.516	2.868	85.970
11	0.462	2.565	88.534
12	0.440	2.447	90.981
13	0.371	2.059	93.041
14	0.324	1.798	94.838
15	0.314	1.744	96.583
16	0.267	1.481	98.064
17	0.194	1.080	99.144
18	0.154	0.856	100.000

To test the null hypothesis that the original correlation matrix was an identity matrix, we used Bartlett's test. The significance test showed that the R-matrix was not an identity matrix; therefore, there were relationships between the variables included in the analysis. For our data, Bartlett's test was highly significant ($x^2 = 496.9$, with degree of freedom $= 153, p < .001$), and therefore, factor analysis was appropriate.

At this stage, the analysis extracted three factors (Table 3). However, the factor structure was not clear. Three of the items were multidimensional, although they loaded highly (eigenvalues > 0.40) on the emerging core factor; they also loaded on the second and third factor. These items were either 12-step specific (e.g., "I am in contact with my sponsor" and "I am sponsoring others") or related to one's family rather than to the individual recovery (e.g., "I encourage my family members to participate in recovery events"). Removing these items from the scale meant that a powerful unidimensional scale could be achieved, where the single factor could be unequivocally interpreted as personal recovery.

Stage 2: 15-Item Version

In PCA on the 15-item scale, a one-factor solution emerged, based on the Birmingham sample. In a subsequent analysis using the same statistical approach, this result was replicated with the total Glasgow sample as well as with two relevant subsamples (Table 4). The explained variance was higher in the Glasgow (67.4%) than in the Birmingham sample (39.3%).

TABLE 3 Loadings of the Variable on the Factors

No.	RGPS item	Factor F1	Factor F2	Factor F3
1	I perform service at meetings.	.744		
2	If I didn't make a meeting at home, the number of people who would call would be . . .	.730		
3	I socialize before or after meeting.	.721		
4	I carry a message of hope to others.	.713		
5	I carry a recovery object.	.671		
6	I attend recovery social events.	.657		
7	I speak at meetings.	.649		
8	I read recovery-supportive literature.	.645		−.427
9	I use daily rituals.	.611	−.418	
10	I attend recovery meetings.	.579		−.467
11	I acknowledge my recovery status.	.570		.493
12	The number of phone numbers of people who support my recovery is . . .	.552		
13	The number of groups I attend regularly is . . .	.501	−.485	
14	I am sponsoring others.		.667	
15	I encourage my family members to participate in recovery events.		.622	
16	I visit a recovery clubhouse.	.467	.514	
17	I do voluntary service in the community.	.496		.504
18	I am in contact with my sponsor.		.435	.539

TABLE 4 PCA of the 15-Item RGPS

No.	RGPS item	Birmingham sample (heroin)	Glasgow total sample	Glasgow subsample former alcohol problems	Glasgow subsample former heroin problems
1	I attend recovery group meetings.	.590	.853	.752	.923
2	The number of groups that I attend regularly is . . .	.537	.824	.724	.923
3	If I did not make a meeting at my home group for 2 weeks, I think the number of people who would call to see if I was OK would be . . .	.716	.859	.780	.919
4	I speak at meetings.	.633	.917	.870	.949
5	I perform service at meetings.	.763	.880	.841	.906
6	I carry a message of hope to others.	.702	.884	.857	.905
7	I socialize before or after meetings.	.722	.904	.849	.945
8	I attend recovery social events.	.642	.814	.737	.869
9	I visit a recovery clubhouse.	.418	.404	.310	.531
10	I read recovery-supportive literature.	.649	.859	.795	.907
11	I carry a recovery object.	.692	.747	.686	.847
12	The number of phone numbers of people who support my recovery is . . .	.582	.918	.876	.948
13	I use daily rituals.	.621	.847	.793	.884
14	I do voluntary service in the community.	.475	.731	.665	.796
15	I acknowledge my recovery status.	.557	.735	.694	.752
	Explained variance	39.3%	67.4%	57.5%	76.2%
	n	219	205	107	98
	Mean (SD)	1.5 (0.6)	1.3 (1.0)	1.5 (0.9)	1.1 (1.1)
	Age (mean; DS)	32.8; 7.6	43.2; 10.9	48.9; 10.8	36.9; 6.9
	Gender (male)	166 (76.1%)	137 (66.8%)	65 (60.7%)	72 (73.5%)

Means were calculated for each sample population (Table 4), and normative data are presented here for all members of each sample or subsample. A t-test performed on the Glasgow data indicated that recovery group participation was significantly higher for the subgroups of participants who were self-reporting abstinence for all psychoactive substances (including prescribed substitute medication) than in the medicated sample (abstinent subgroup mean = 1.5±0.6 vs. medicated subgroup mean = 0.7±0.8), $t =$ 4.17, $p <$ .0001). This finding supports the validity of the scale because previous research has indicated that recovery group participation is significantly positively related to abstinence (for reviews, see Humphreys, 2004; Humphreys et al., 2004; Kelly & Yeterian, 2008; White, 2009). Analysis of the Birmingham data, however, did not show significant differences between the mean scores of the abstinent and maintained groups.

Associations With RGPS Total Score

To assess the consistency of the 15-item scale with other linked measures, correlation analysis was conducted between the RGPS total score and measures of current functioning and of social networks, as reported in Table 5.

There were statistically significant associations between the RGPS total score and three of the four measures of quality of life—psychological, social, and lived environment—and with number of nonusers in recovery and time spent with nonusers in recovery. Higher RGPS scores were also associated with higher levels of reported self-esteem but not with self-efficacy.

DISCUSSION

While there are a number of scales that measure the extent of 12-step and AA affiliation, there are no generic measures of engagement in nonaffiliated

TABLE 5 Association Between RGPS Total Score and Measures of Current Functioning

Current functioning and social networks measure	R coefficient	Significance
Physical quality of life	.08	.20
Psychological quality of life	.17	.02
Social quality of life	.24	.001
Quality of Life Living environment	.29	.001
Self-esteem	.15	.03
Self-efficacy	.05	.50
Numbers of nonusers in social network	.07	.34
Numbers of users in recovery in social network	.44	.001
Numbers of current users	.08	.29
Time (in mins) spent with nonusers	−.14	.06
Time (in mins) spent with nonusers in recovery	.37	.001
Time (in mins) spent with users	−.15	.11

recovery groups. The current measure was designed to incorporate not only 12-step engagement but engagement with other mutual aid organizations, such as SMART recovery and nontherapeutic recovery groups, including those linked to vocational or interest groups where people in recovery meet to provide each other with mutual support.

The initial scaling was assessed using a sample from Birmingham consisting of individuals typically in the early stages of their recovery journey, including those in "service user groups" linked to treatment and prescribing services. From this analysis, a two-factor model was derived and reduced to a single factor scale that focused on engagement to the exclusion of a secondary factor that related more to family involvement in recovery groups.

This 15-item scale was then reassessed with a mixed group of alcohol and drug users in recovery from a second sample (from Glasgow) with a strong single factor in both of these recovery populations. Furthermore, the total score from this scale was associated with both reported social networks and indicators of current functioning. Thus, individuals with greater engagement in recovery groups reported better self-esteem and higher scores on three of the four scales of quality of life measured by the World Health Organization Quality of Life Brief scale. It is noticeable that there were particularly strong relationships with social and environmental quality of life, which suggests that greater engagement in recovery groups is linked to more satisfactory perceptions of social networks and more satisfactory engagement in the local community and the lived environment.

However, these data are cross-sectional, and it would require longitudinal research to establish the causal linkages between participation in a range of collective recovery activities and quality of life and functioning. Furthermore, the mean scale scores reported were typically low—averaging between 1 and 2 out of 15—and so the associations with functioning at higher levels of recovery group participation remain untested. These low mean scale scores also suggest typically low levels of recovery group participation in UK samples. Also, in the absence of longitudinal data, it is not clear the extent to which recovery group participation provides some kind of protective effect against relapse.

While there is an established evidence base that shows 12-step participation is linked to better outcomes (e.g., Laudet, 2007), this association for generic recovery group activity is as yet untested and is particularly important as we start to assess the role of recovery group supports in medication-maintained drug treatments. However, in locations in which there is greater skepticism about AA and 12-step, such as in the United Kingdom (e.g., Day, Gaston, Furlong, Murali, & Copello, 2005), a broader measure of recovery group engagement may be useful. We are encouraged by the potential benefit of the RGPS to research in the field of addiction recovery and assess and compare disparate interventions (e.g., SMART recovery vs. 12-step model in the future).

The 15-item RGPS offers a rapid assessment technique for assessing engagement in recovery activities that can be used as part of recovery assessment and monitoring and which can be incorporated within a "strengths-based" recovery framework for supporting long-term recovery pathways. Its brief and easy-to-administer format means that it can be used in conjunction with other measures of functioning, such as the Addiction Severity Index and other recovery indicators, including 12-step affiliation measures. However, it offers the opportunity to assess community engagement and the need for assertive linkage that may be valuable in a range of clinical and recovery support settings.

REFERENCES

Barrett, P., & Kline, P. (1981). The observation to variable ratio in factor analyses. *Journal of Personality and Group Behavior, 1*, 23–33.

Best, D., Day, E., Cantillano, V., Gaston, R. L., Nambamali, A., Sweeting, R., & Keaney, F. (2008). Mapping heroin careers: Utilizing a standardized history-taking method to assess the speed of escalation of heroin-using careers in a treatment-seeking cohort. *Drug and Alcohol Review, 27*(2), 165–170.

Best, D., Gow, J., Knox, T., Taylor, A., Groshkova, T., & White, W. (in press). Mapping the recovery stories of drinkers and drug users in Glasgow: Quality of life and its predictors. *Drug and Alcohol Review*. Manuscript submitted for publication.

Best, D., & Groshkova, T. (2011). The assessment of recovery capital: Properties and psychometrics of a measure of recovery strengths and threats. Manuscript in preparation.

Best, D., Groshkova, T., Sadler, J., Day, E., & White, W. (in press). The recovery experiences of a service user group and their peer networks in Birmingham, England. *Alcoholism Treatment Quarterly*. Manuscript submitted for publication.

Bond, J., Kaskutas, L. A., & Weisner, C. (2003). The persistent influence of social networks and Alcoholics Anonymous on abstinence. *Journal of Studies on Alcohol, 64*(4), 579–588.

Cacciola, J. S., Dugosh, K., Foltz, C., Leahy, P., & Stevens, R. (2005). Treatment outcomes: First-time versus treatment-experienced clients. *Journal of Substance Abuse Treatment, 28*, S13–S22.

Connors, G. J., & Dermen, K. H. (1996). Characteristics of participants in Secular Organization for Sobriety. *American Journal of Alcohol and Drug Abuse, 19*(4), 281–295.

Day, E., Best, D., Cantillano, V., Gaston, R., Nambamali, A., & Keaney, F. (2008). Measuring the use and career histories of drug users in treatment: Reliability of the Lifetime Drug Use History (LDUH) and its data yield relative to clinical case notes. *Drug and Alcohol Review, 27*(2), 171–177.

Day, E., Gaston, R. L., Furlong, E., Murali, V., & Copello, A. (2005). United Kingdom substance misuse treatment workers' attitudes toward 12-step self-help groups. *Journal of Substance Abuse Treatment, 29*(4), 321–327.

Dennis, M. L., Titus, J. C., White, M. K., Unsicker, J. I., & Hodgkins, D. (2002). *Global appraisal of individual needs: Administration guide for the GAIN and related measures*. Bloomington, IL: Chestnut Health Systems, Lighthouse Institute. Retrieved from http://www.chestnut.org/li/gain

Emrick, C., Tonigan, J. S., Montgomery, H., & Little, L. (1993). Alcoholics Anonymous: What is currently known? In B. S. McCrady & W. R. Miller (Eds.), *Research on Alcoholics Anonymous: Opportunities and alternatives* (pp. 41–76). New Brunswick, NJ: Rutgers.

Gilbert, F. S. (1991). Development of a "Steps Questionnaire." *Journal of Studies on Alcohol, 52*, 353–360.

Hillhouse, M. P., & Fiorentine, R. (2001). 12-step program participation and effectiveness: Do gender and ethnic differences exist? *Journal of Drug Issues, 31*(3), 767–780.

Horvath, A. (1999/2000). SMART recovery. *International Journal of Self-Help and Self-Care, 1*(2), 163–169.

Humphreys, K. (2003). Alcohol and drug abuse: A research-based analysis of the moderation management controversy. *Psychiatric Services, 54*, 621–622.

Humphreys, K. (2004). *Circles of recovery: Self-help organizations for addictions.* Cambridge, United Kingdom: Cambridge University Press.

Humphreys, K. (2006). The trial of Alcoholics Anonymous. *Addiction, 101*, 617–618.

Humphreys, K., Kaskutas, L., & Weisner, C. (1998). The Alcoholics Anonymous Affiliation Scale: Development, reliability, and norms for diverse treated and untreated populations. *Alcoholism: Clinical and Experimental Research, 22*(5), 974–978.

Humphreys, K., & Klaw, E. (2001). Can targeting nondependent problem drinkers and providing Internet-based services expand access to assistance for alcohol problems? A study of the Moderation Management self-help/mutual aid organization. *Journal of Studies on Alcohol, 62*(4), 528–532.

Humphreys, K., Moos, R. J., & Cohen, C. (1997). Social and community resources and long-term recovery from treated and untreated alcoholism. *Journal of Studies on Alcohol, 58*(3), 231–238.

Humphreys, K., & Moos, R. H. (1996). Reduced substance-related health care costs among voluntary participants in Alcoholics Anonymous. *Psychiatric Services, 47*(7), 709–713.

Humphreys, K., & Moos, R. H. (2001). Can encouraging substance abuse patients to participate in self-help groups reduce demand for health care? A quasiexperimental study. *Alcoholism: Clinical and Experimental Research, 255*, 711–716.

Humphreys, K., Moos, R. J., & Cohen, C. (1997). Social and community resources and long-term recovery from treated and untreated alcoholism. *Journal of Studies on Alcohol, 58*(3), 231–238.

Humphreys, K., Wing, S., McCarty, D., Chappel, J., Galant, L., Haberle, B., . . . Weiss, R. (2004). Self-help organizations for alcohol and drug problems: Toward evidence-based practice and policy. *Journal of Substance Abuse Treatment, 26*(3), 151–158.

Joe, G. W., Broome, K. M., Rowan-Szal, G. A., & Simpson, D. D. (2002). Measuring patient attributes and engagement in treatment. *Journal of Substance Abuse Treatment, 22*(4), 183–196.

Jolliffe, I. T. (2002). *Principal component analysis* (2nd ed., Springer Series in Statistics). New York, NY: Springer-Verlag New York.

Kaskutas, L. A. (2009). Alcoholics Anonymous effectiveness: Faith meets science. *Journal of Addictive Diseases, 28*, 145–157.

Kaskutas, L. A., Ammon, L. N., Delucchi, K., Room, R., Bond, J., & Weisner, C. (2005). Alcoholics Anonymous careers: Patterns of AA involvement 5 years after treatment entry. *Alcoholism: Clinical and Experimental Research, 29*(11), 1983–1990.

Kaskutas, L. A., Subbaraman, M., Witbrodt, J., & Zemore, S. (2009). Effectiveness of Making Alcoholics Anonymous Easier (MAAEZ), a group-format 12-step facilitation approach. *Journal of Substance Abuse Treatment, 37*(3), 228–239.

Kelly, J. F., Myers, M. G., & Brown, S. A. (2002). A multivariate process model of adolescent 12-step attendance and substance use outcome following inpatient treatment. *Psychology of Addictive Behaviors, 14*, 376–389.

Kelly, J. F., & Yeterian, J. (2008). Mutual-help groups. In W. O'Donohue & J. R. Cunningham (Eds.), *Evidence-based adjunctive treatments* (pp. 61–106). New York, NY: Elsevier.

Kline, P. (2000). A psychometrics primer. London, United Kingdom: Free Association Books.

Kownacki, R. J., & Shadish, W. R. (1999). Does Alcoholics Anonymous work? The results from a meta-analysis of controlled experiments. *Substance Use and Misuse, 34*(13), 1897–1916.

Laudet, A. B. (2007). What does recovery mean to you? Lessons from the recovery experience for research and practice. *Journal of Substance Abuse Treatment, 33*, 243–256.

Laudet, A. B., Cleland, C. M., Magura, S., Vogel, H. S., & Knight, E. L. (2004). Social support mediates the effects of dual-focus mutual-aid groups on abstinence from substance use. *American Journal of Community Psychology, 34*, 175–185.

Longabaugh, R., Wirtz, P. W., Zweben, A., & Stout, R. L. (1998). Network support for drinking: Alcoholics Anonymous and long-term matching efforts. *Addiction, 93*, 1313–1333.

Montgomery, H. A., Miller, W. R., & Tonigan, J. S. (1995). Does Alcoholics Anonymous involvement predict treatment outcome? *Journal of Substance Abuse Treatment, 12*(4), 241–246.

Moos, R. H. (2008). Active ingredients of substance use-focused self-help groups. *Addiction, 103*, 387–396.

Moos, R. H., & Moos, B. S. (2004). Help-seeking careers: Connections between participation in professional treatment and Alcoholics Anonymous. *Journal of Substance Abuse Treatment, 26*, 167–173.

Morgenstern, J., Kahler, C. W., Frey, R. M., & Labouvie, E. (1996). Modeling therapeutic response to 12-step treatment: Optimal responders, nonresponders, partial responders. *Journal of Substance Abuse, 8*(1), 45–59.

Morgenstern, J., Labouvie, E., McCray, B. S., Kahler, C. W., & Frey, R. M. (1997). Affiliation with Alcoholics Anonymous after treatment: A study of its therapeutic effects and mechanisms of action. *Journal of Consulting and Clinical Psychology, 65*(5), 768–777.

Munro, B. H. (2001). *Statistical methods for health care research.* Philadelphia, PA: Lippincott.

Nunnally, J. C., & Bernstein, I. H. (1994). *Psychometric theory* (3rd ed.). New York, NY: McGraw-Hill.

Roman, P. M., & Blum, T. C. (1997). National treatment center study. Athens, GA: Institute of Behavioral Research, University of Georgia.

Sheeren, M. (1988). The relationship between relapse and involvement in Alcoholics Anonymous. *Journal of Studies on Alcohol, 49*(1), 104–106.

Tonigan, J., Connors, G., & Miller, W. (1996). Alcoholics Anonymous Involvement (AAI) scale: Reliability and norms. *Psychology of Addictive Behaviors, 10,* 75–80.

Tonigan, J. S., Toscova, R., & Miller, W. R. (1996). Meta-analysis of the literature on Alcoholics Anonymous: Sample and study characteristics moderate findings. *Journal of Studies on Alcohol, 57*(1), 65–72.

Toumbourou, J. W., Hamilton, M., U'Ren, A., Stevens-Jones, P., & Storey, G. (2002). Narcotics Anonymous participation and changes in substance use and social support. *Journal of Substance Abuse Treatment, 23,* 61–66.

West, R. (1991). *Computing for psychologists.* London, England: Harwood Academic.

White, W. (1998). *Slaying the dragon: The history of addiction treatment and recovery in America.* Bloomington, IL: Chestnut Health Systems/Lighthouse Institute.

White, W. (2004). Addiction recovery mutual-aid groups: An enduring international phenomenon. *Addiction, 99,* 532–538.

White, W. (2009). *Peer-based addiction recovery support: History, theory, practice, and scientific evaluation.* Chicago, IL: Great Lakes Addiction Technology Transfer Center and Philadelphia Department of Behavioral Health and Mental Retardation Services.

White, W., & Gasperin, D. (2006). *Addiction treatment and recovery: A primer for criminal justice personnel.* Springfield, IL: University of Illinois–Springfield Center for Legal and Policy Studies.

White, W., & Kurtz, E. (2006). The varieties of recovery experience. *International Journal of Self-Help and Self-Care, 3*(1/2), 21–61.

White, W., & Nicolaus, M. (2005). Styles of secular recovery. *Counselor, 6*(4), 58–61.

World Health Organization. (1993). *WHOQOL study protocol (MNH 7PSF/93.9), 1993.* Geneva, Switzerland: Author.

World Health Organization Quality of Life Group. (1998a). Development of the World Health Organization WHOQOL-BREF quality of life assessment. *Psychological Medicine, 28*(3), 551–558.

World Health Organization Quality of Life Group. (1998b). The World Health Organization Quality of Life Assessment: Development and general psychometric properties. *Social Science and Medicine, 46*(12), 1569–1585.

Zemore, S. E., Kaskutas, L. E., & Ammon, L. N. (2004). In 12-step groups, helping helps the helper. *Addiction, 99,* 1015–1023.

APPENDIX: FINAL RGPS VERSION

		(0)	(1)	(2)	(3)
1.	I attend recovery group meetings.	Never	1-2 times per week	3-4 times per week	5 or more times per week
2.	The number of groups that I attend regularly is. . .	None	One	2-4	5 or more
3.	If I did not make a meeting at my home group for 2 weeks, I think the number of people who would call to see if I was OK would be. . .	None	One	2-4	5 or more
4.	I speak at meetings.	Never	Rarely	Sometimes	Frequently
5.	I perform service at meetings.	Never	Rarely	Sometimes	Frequently
6.	I carry a message of hope to others.	Never	Rarely	Sometimes	Frequently
7.	I socialize before or after meetings.	Never	Rarely	Sometimes	Frequently
8.	I attend recovery social events.	Never	Rarely	Sometimes	Frequently
9.	I visit a recovery clubhouse.	Never	Rarely	Sometimes	Frequently
10.	I read recovery supportive literature.	Never	Rarely	Sometimes	Frequently
11.	I carry a recovery object.	Never	Rarely	Sometimes	Frequently
12.	The number of phone numbers of people who support my recovery is. . .	None	1-5	6-9	10 or more
13.	I use daily rituals.	Never	Rarely	Sometimes	Frequently
14.	I do voluntary service in the community.	Never	Rarely	Sometimes	Frequently
15.	I acknowledge my recovery status.	Never	Rarely	Sometimes	Frequently

Community Rehabilitation in the United Kingdom—What Place Does It Have?

MARION LOGAN

Director of Operations—Scotland, Phoenix Futures, Glasgow, Scotland, United Kingdom

It has long been established that having a range of treatment options readily available within a given geographical area is a minimum requirement for effective outcomes to be achieved by those affected by problematic substance misuse. This is recognized within national strategy documents, namely, the Scottish Government's The Road to Recovery and the UK Government's Drugs: Protecting Families and Communities (The Home Office, 2008), in numerous reports and within local partnerships' strategy documents. Indeed the core message of the Essential Care publication (The Scottish Government, 2008) was to state what the minimum should contain.

A concern of many is the lack of standardization of service provision. Hence, the decision in Scotland in 2005 was to develop national quality standards for substance misuse services, following extensive consultation the standards, and they were published in 2006. However, the concern remains that in some part of the country visiting your pharmacy 6 days per week is the sum total of your "therapeutic engagement." This article proposes a new model for community rehabilitation—one in which the community location and linkage is critical and where meaningful change can occur.

The concept of community rehabilitation has been around for many years. Within Scotland, it is even accorded its own "category" within the Waiting Times database (The Scottish Executive, 2003):

Community based support and/or rehabilitation—Interventions that have the purpose of tackling the social and psychological problems faced by the client (such as debt / benefit / relationship and family problems, relapse prevention or employability and training issues; e.g., structured day [programs], [counseling], group work). Clients may be in receipt of other treatment interventions in parallel with community based support and rehabilitation (e.g., substitute prescribing).

It is this last sentence that has resulted in a distinct shift in recent years. As the number of people in receipt of "substitute prescribing," for methadone in particular, has increased, so the range of provision available has often become narrower.

The rapid development of methadone maintenance prescribing as the "gold standard" treatment often resulted in community rehabilitation programs' identity being subsumed as the program part of the methadone maintenance program.

Many may argue that the decline in the preference for residential rehabilitation was simply a case of the huge increase in the number of problem drug users. However, the reasons behind the shift were as much to do with the change in the sector's view as with the overall purpose of drug treatment. The targets by which the sector was measured focused on how people got to the service; no mention was made of what happened to them once they were there. Until very recently, Governmental emphasis was on access and retention, on the number of new service users, no information was requested about total number of service users in each service or on length of time service users remained with a service. This situation was underpinned by the view that drug dependency should be viewed as a long-term chronic health problem, akin to diabetes. Therefore, substitute prescribing was for life. This, coupled with the view that ready access to a prescription of reasonable dose would help people stay alive and well, reduce drug-related deaths, and help prevent the spread of blood-borne viruses, have all contributed to the loss of understanding as to what a community rehabilitation could offer and the difference it could make.

Then there was recognition that for some people a community-based program was not only more suitable but was actually preferable. However, over time, in many people's minds, community rehabilitation has translated into long-term methadone maintenance with a couple of groups on the side. In some areas and with the support of many clinicians and workers in the field, there is no need for anything other than ready access to a minimum dose of methadone for as long as you want it (Scottish Government, 2007a).

Methadone maintenance, indeed medically supported recovery, should be one of the range of options available; however, it is necessary to ensure that the "prescription" does not dominate or be accorded a more significant role in the recovery process than the other elements, in particular the development of supportive, encouraging relationships (for a discussion of the issues, see Rosier, 2010).

As is clearly stated in the recently published *NHS Scotland HEAT Performance Management System 2009–10 TARGET A11—To offer drug misusers faster access to appropriate treatment to support their recovery* (The Scottish Government, 2009),

> . . . although important, substitute prescribing on its own is not enough, nor should it be seen as the only option for treatment of opiate users.

We know from numerous research studies that a key contributing factor in an individual's successful recovery journey is the quality of the relationships they build with those offering help and support (Najavits, Crits-Christoph, & Dierberger, 2000; Project Match Research Group, 1999; White, 2008). In the United Kingdom, this significant feature has over time been systematically ignored by commissioners and forgotten or downplayed by workers in the field. In recent years, some providers, often in response to increased demand, have shortened the amount of actual meaningful contact time in the belief that the effectiveness of the program will be unaffected. Wrong. The result is a service that focuses on containment, not recovery. When you have clinicians and commissioners believing that contact with a key worker and building a 1-to-1 relationship can be replaced by attendance at a "monitoring clinic" for 10 minutes every 6 weeks to no detrimental effect, you have to wonder whether "recovery" as a defining concept has lost all meaning.

So how can we rectify the situation? Initially, we need to challenge any possible misunderstanding brilliantly exemplified in the following question that was asked in a recent consultation document from the Scottish Government:

> Residential Rehabilitation and Structured Day [Programs]: there are questions around whether these interventions are fundamentally different in nature (i.e., are they effectively the same range of interventions, merely delivered in two different settings?). Should they be represented by a single treatment modality? Information Statistics Division (ISD Scotland) and the Scottish Government are frequently asked about the numbers of people waiting for residential rehabilitation as opposed to those waiting for community-based support of one kind or another, so from a data analysis point of view, this is a useful distinction. Possibly less so from a clinical perspective, so would it be useful to make this explicit in our descriptions of the modalities? (Scottish Government, 2010)

There are and should be huge differences between a residential rehabilitation program and a structured day program—however, it should also be acknowledged that just because someone is in a residential setting does not mean they are benefitting from a rehabilitation program. One critical factor as stated above is how much time is structured. For example, a structured day program that only requires an individual to participate for a couple of hours a day for only 3 days per week is a different concept from a 5-day-a-week, 6-hour-a-day program. Also, some so-called residential programs have little structured activity (e.g., one group per day plus one mutual aid group). The amount of structured time and the corresponding requirement for the individual to actively demonstrate their commitment to participating in the program is another deciding factor. It is as interesting to ask under what circumstances someone would be asked to leave, as it is to ask what the eligibility criteria is for access.

Therefore, within our understanding of community rehabilitation, there should be a minimum time element, or else one person's community rehabil-itation is another's psychosocial intervention—an agreed goal, an emphasis on progress, and an endpoint.

Key issues that such services need to address are accessibility, frequency of contact, and intensity of program (Scottish Government, 2007b). We need to reeducate the field and indeed the general public that community-based rehabilitation programs are one of the ranges of appropriate treatment and rehabilitation services that must be available at a local level. However, the emphasis of these services is on supporting individuals on their recovery journey, not on retaining treatment for the sake of retention. As Bill White explained, is the individual "working on their recovery," thus the support from the service being understood as a milestone in their recovery career, or are they "doing time" and is their attendance at the service being understood as a "milestone in their addiction career" (Phoenix House USA Consultation Questions & Responses, personal communication, 2009)?

Reviews of the effectiveness of any treatment intervention highlight sev-eral essential components, namely speed and ease of access, relationship between worker and service user—sometimes referred to as "therapeutic alliance"—and on-going proactive contact (personal communication, Bill White and Phoenix House USA, 2009).

For community rehabilitation programs to meaningfully contribute to an individual's recovery journey, the balance between the variables (as shown in Table 1) needs to be discussed and agreed upon. It is important to emphasize that these variables are not to be understood as an either/or but as on a continuum. However this does not apply to specifying at the outset the intended outcome of the support. A service that tries to meet the needs of those with different goals can struggle to meet the needs of anyone. In the views of many service users and indeed staff, providing a service for those with different goals can be an unsatisfactory experience for all.

Once this is done, the most important step is to then communicate exactly who the service is for, what difference it will make, and how it

TABLE 1 Intervention Program Criteria Variables

Open	Closed
Minimum Attendance	User defined
Staged Program	Flexible
Core Elements	No core requirements
Endpoint	Indefinite attendance
Staff led	Peer led
Separate program	Integrated with other interventions
Therapeutic	Vocational
Task centered	Process focus
Certificated elements	Noncertified
Mixed Gender	Single Gender
Abstinence Focus	Harm Reduction

fits with other options available. In commissioner terms, this is the service specification, the performance measures, inputs, outputs, and outcomes.

A key requirement for community rehabilitation programs is that they have strong, sustainable links within the community in which they are based. The service and the staff need to view themselves as a resource, as a facilitator of change, as a contact point, and most importantly, as a stage in people lives, not the main feature. In reality, the most successful community rehabilitation programs need to have "employment/training or voluntary work" as a key performance indicator. As much research (Best et al., 2008; Day et al., 2008; McKeganey, Bloor, McIntosh, & Neale, 2008) has demonstrated, engagement in "meaningful activity" is a key factor in maintaining recovery goals.

The focus of much activity within Scotland—and in the rest of the United Kingdom—has been on improving access (Home Office, 2008). Clearly, as a performance measure, having services that are readily accessible is an important indicator, but it is not the only one. In Scotland, the developments of waiting times will see a shift from calculating wait from a service perspective to calculating wait from a service user's perspective. Ultimately, it is the Scottish Government's "aim that all drug treatment services, no matter who they are funded by, will work to ensure that people with drug problems get access to the treatment they need within 3 weeks of referral" (The Scottish Government, 2010).

In an ideal world, no one would wait for the help they need. We do not live in an ideal world. Nor, until recently, have we had a serious debate about the purpose of drug rehabilitation services. If, as is being widely stated, it is about recovery—and recovery as understood to encompass the absence of problematic substance use (in many cases, abstinence), improvement in global (physical and mental) health, and positive participation in and contribution to community life (White, 2009), then we need to start focusing on the "contract" between the service user and the service. This is not about providing a minimal level of service to every problematic drug user. It is about stating, clearly and unemotionally, if you want to change your life and the relationship you have with drugs, this is what we can offer you. If you wanted to continue to take drugs, information is available to try and minimize the harm to yourself and others. The primary focus of a community rehabilitation service should be to engage with those individuals who want to change their lives. There are other models of service delivery available for those individuals who are not yet at the decision stage.

It is some progress that we have explicit statements that there should be a range of services and that work is in progress to improve definitions (see The Scottish Government, 2008). However, it cannot be said that this desire has actually been enforced or progress meaningfully reported. As stated above, there are a number of variables that need to be explored to identify the core components of an effective community rehabilitation service.

Although it is recognized that there have been shifts in perspective during the past few years, the evidence that service provision, staff activity, and beliefs are focused on long-term recovery and promoting this as not only desirable but possible is not readily available in all parts of the United Kingdom. What we do need is to demand such evidence is readily produced and publicly available. In the face of severe public sector cuts, there has never been a better reason to get our house in order. The UK Government wants a public debate on what should be provided by the government and what services/activities can be more effectively provided by other types of organizations:

> Every spending [program] would face 'probing questions,' he said—including whether it was essential, could be done cheaper or could be delivered by the private or voluntary sector. (BBC, 2010)

This is our opportunity to demonstrate what community-based rehabilitation services should be funded, what those services should be designed to provide, and the criteria by which their impact should be measured.

A question that has been asked a number of times since the shift in focus to recovery-orientated services in the United Kingdom is, "Can we afford recovery?" The only sensible response to this is "Can we afford not to have that as our focus?"

Much mention is made of not having a "one size fits all" approach. However, neither should we have a "lowest common denominator" approach to service provision. The key is in the use of the word "engagement"; why fund and provide a service that people do not want or do not want to engage with? We need to provide services that make a difference and for which we can readily demonstrate the difference they make.

There is a real need to develop different "models" of service delivery within the substance misuse sector. In the United Kingdom, the key (in this author's opinion) is on ceasing to be quite so isolationist and truly embrace the recovery concept, not by changing the name of the service but by changing the basis of how the workers and managers interact with service users and whole operational methodology. In essence, this is about becoming the community resource. It requires the guiding principle to be for workers to understand themselves and their role as one of facilitator, not expert. The path to recovery is an individual one, but it is rarely done alone or in isolation for the rest of someone's life. Individuals will go through similar stages and require the same types of support; the pace of progress and intensity of support will of course vary, and this is why we need flexible, responsive support.

During the past 2 years, Phoenix Futures UK has developed a service model that encompasses the importance of strong community links and recognizes that support for recovery is about more than cessation of problematic drug/alcohol use and that support needs vary from individual to individual and over time.

Our recovery HUB model operates successfully in both cities and rural areas. It is characterized by greater flexibility in opening times, draws on the knowledge and expertise of a range of other organizations, and promotes recovery as a visible, achievable goal for all. By developing formal partnerships with a range of other organizations, we are able to increase understanding of the effects of addiction and to reduce the stigma of seeking help. This also enables recovery HUBs to be as beneficial to the family members as to the individual services user.

The funding arrangements for all tax-payer-funded services in the United Kingdom are going through a difficult, uncertain time. Now, more than ever, we need to be very clear what we are providing and what difference it makes.

REFERENCES

BBC. (2010, June 8). *Osborne to consult public about spending choices.* Retrieved from http://news.bbc.co.uk/1/hi/politics/10261136.stm

Best, D., Day, E., Cantillano, V., Gaston, R., Nambamali, A., Sweeting, R., & Keaney, F. (2008). Mapping heroin careers: Utilizing a standardized history-taking method to assess the speed of escalation of heroin-using careers in a treatment-seeking cohort. *Drug and Alcohol Review, 27,* 169–174.

Day, E., Best, D., Cantillano, V., Gaston, V., Nambamali, A., & Keaney, F. (2008). Measuring the use and career histories of drug users in treatment: Reliability of the Lifetime Drug Use History (LDUH) and its data yield relative to clinical case notes. *Drug and Alcohol Review, 27,* 175–181.

The Home Office. (2008). *Drugs: Protecting families and communities.* Retrieved from http://webarchive.nationalarchives.gov.uk/20100419081707/drugs.homeoffice.gov.uk/publication-search/drug-strategy/drug-strategy-2008.html

McKeganey, N., Bloor, M., McIntosh, J., & Neale J. (2008). *Key findings from the Drug Outcome Research in Scotland (DORIS) Study* (Center for Drug Misuse Research Occasional Paper). Glasgow, Scotland: University of Glasgow.

Najavits, L. M., Crits-Christoph, P., & Dierberger, A. (2000). Clinicians' impact on the quality of substance use disorder treatment. *Substance Use and Misuse, 35*(12), 2161–2190.

Project MATCH Research Group. (1999). Summary of Project MATCH. *Addiction, 94*(1), 31–34.

Rosier, M. (2010, April 24). Medication-assisted recovery—Emerging trends in the treatment of substance use disorders. *The Counselor, 11*(2). Retrieved from http://www.counselormagazine.com/home?func=show_edition&id=24

Schering-Plough. (2008). *The management of drug dependency in Scotland: More than methadone?* For more information, e-mail norma.nicholl@spcorp.com

The Scottish Executive. (2003). *National waiting times framework. Retrieved from* http://www.drugmisuse.isdscotland.org/wtpilot/Framework.pdf

The Scottish Government. (2007a). *Reducing harm and promoting recovery: A report on methadone treatment for substance misuse in Scotland.* Retrieved from http://www.scotland.gov.uk/publications/2007/06/22094730/0

The Scottish Government. (2007b). *Review of methadone in drug treatment: Prescribing information and practice.* Retrieved from http://www.scotland.gov.uk/publications/2007/06/22094632/1

The Scottish Government. (2008). *Essential care: —A report on the approach required to maximize opportunity for recovery from problem substance use in Scotland.* Retrieved from http://www.scotland.gov.uk/Publications/2008/03/20144059/0

The Scottish Government. (2009). *NHS Scotland HEAT Performance Management System 2009–10 TARGET A11—To offer drug misusers faster access to appropriate treatment to support their recovery: Guidance on referral pathway.* Retrieved from http://www.scotland.gov.uk/resource/doc/254430/0097982.pdf

The Scottish Government. (2010a). *A wait off our shoulders: A guide to improving access to recovery-focused drug and alcohol treatment services in Scotland.* Retrieved from http://www.scotland.gov.uk/Resource/Doc/313876/0099592.pdf

The Scottish Government. (2010b). HEAT Technical Support Group Consultation on the definition of treatment modalities for drug and alcohol interventions. Retrieved from http://www.drugmisuse.isdscotland.org/wtpilot/DATWT_TreatmentTypes_rev.pdf

White W. L. (2008). *Recovery management and recovery-oriented systems of care: Scientific rationale and promising practices.* Pittsburgh, PA: Northeast Addiction Technology Transfer Center, The Great Lakes Addiction Technology Transfer Center, and the Philadelphia Department of Behavioral Health/Mental Retardation Services. Retrieved from http://www.attcnetwork.org/userfiles/file/GreatLakes/mng993-DLD1.pdf

White, W. (2009). *Peer-based addiction recovery support: History, theory, practice, and scientific evaluation.* Chicago, IL: Great Lakes Addiction Technology Transfer Center and Philadelphia Department of Behavioral Health and Mental Retardation Services.

Therapeutic Communities: *Can-Do* Attitudes for *Must-Have* Recovery

ROWDY YATES

Scottish Addiction Studies, Department of Applied Social Sciences, University of Stirling, Stirling, Scotland, United Kingdom

The therapeutic community (TC) in the United Kingdom was built out of a merging of the democratic TC tradition pioneered by Maxwell Jones and others immediately after the Second World War and after the American drug-free TC originating in the Synanon experiment in the late 1950s. This latter tradition traces its roots back through the mutual-aid fellowship Alcoholics Anonymous (AA). This article examines how AA principles were adapted for the TC and how this new approach impacted upon the early drug treatment network in the United Kingdom. The evidence base for TC methodology is briefly described along with a short analysis of the marginalization of the approach in the past two decades and the future possibilities for modified TCs for special populations.

THERAPEUTIC COMMUNITIES: A SHORT HISTORY

The roots of the modern drug-free therapeutic community (TC) movement lie in the mutual-aid fellowship Alcoholics Anonymous (AA; Broekaert, Vandervelde, Soyez, Yates, & Slater, 2006; De Leon, 1997; Rawlings & Yates, 2001), which, in its turn, was the continuation of a long history of self-help recovery groups including the Washingtonians, the Jacoby Clubs, and the Blue Cross (Fédération Internationale de la Croix-Bleue; White, 2000; Yates & Malloch, 2010). In its early years, the TC attracted the interest and support of many medical practitioners and academics, and in Europe in particular, this led to a merging of TC practice with the social psychiatry innovations of Jones, Laing, Clarke, Mandelbrote, Basaglia, and others. This earlier European tradition of "democratic" TCs within the developing social psychiatry tradition (Clarke, 2003; Kennard, 1983; Vandevelde, 1999) both ensured the acceptance of the new addiction TCs and served to temper some of their more antitreatment attitudes (Kooyman, 1992; Ravndal, 2003; Rawlings & Yates, 2001). Indeed, in Europe, most addiction TCs were initially established by enthusiastic psychiatrists. However, despite this apparently ready acceptance within addiction psychiatry circles, it is equally true that TCs—and the mutual-aid fellowships from which they sprang—have continued to be viewed with some suspicion by many within mainstream addiction treatment (Best, 2010; Best, Harris, & Strang, 2000). In part, this seems to be a natural consequence of a traditional, infection control-focused view of substance use disorders as a phenomenon to be managed and contained. But in part also, it appears to stem from a concern that TCs have failed to establish evidential credentials in a field increasingly dominated by the demand for evidence-based treatments.

The drug-free TC, or "concept house," began with Charles Dederich's *Synanon* experiment in a derelict waterfront hotel in Santa Monica, CA, in 1958 (Rawlings & Yates, 2001; Yablonsky, 1965). While Synanon had grown out of Dederich's experiences as a member of AA for a number of years, he and his fellow travelers had identified two critical elements missing from the 12-step program, which they felt were necessary for successful recovery from heroin addiction. Firstly, because most of the heroin addicts they were dealing with had little experience of the work environment, they recognized that this particular group would need a more intensive intervention that combined therapy with a structured work program. Secondly, they had grown increasingly restless at AA's insistence on not challenging the individual's own story, or "cross talking" as it was then termed. Dederich and his fellow adventurers felt that there were numerous times when a fellow recoveree needed to be told, in no uncertain terms, that they were rationalizing their behavior or sugar-coating an unpalatable truth. It was out of these two beliefs that Synanon developed as a hierarchical structured program revolving around the "Game," an uninhibited maelstrom of verbal condemnation, insult, and abuse, later to be rebadged by Carl Rogers as the "encounter group" (Yates, 2003).

Bassin (1978) has described the despair that many professionals were feeling during that period, at the failure of existing treatment programs to do more than "contain the whirlwind" of destruction that howled around the drug addict. Although some research (Robins & Murphy, 1967; Winick, 1962) pointed to a natural "maturing out" of addicts in their 30s, there was little hope that existing treatment practice could achieve more than a minimal impact on the dramatic increases in levels of addiction.

America's major treatment facilities were recording depressingly high levels of relapse. Figures show that the relapse rate for the Riverside Hospital in New York was almost 100% (Vaillant, 1966), while in the much-vaunted methadone experiment at the Rockefeller University Hospital in New York (Dole & Nyswander, 1965), almost 20% of those in the program for 6 months or more had been arrested; and this was found despite a screening process that rejected approximately 50% of volunteers to the program as being "unmotivated." Indeed, with a less rigid selection criteria, in a similar experiment in Canada, of 321 addicts recruited, a remarkable 264 (82%) dropped out of the program (Louria, 1968).

So the news that a group of ex-heroin addicts in California appeared to have stumbled onto the ingredients of a successful "cure" was greeted with excitement in some quarters and sheer incredulity in others. It was not long before a series of communities had been established using basic Synanon principles and often Synanon graduates. Phoenix House in New York and Daytop Village (Drug Addicts Treated on Probation) on Staten Island were among the first communities, and the movement quickly blossomed across the United States and was transposed to Europe (Broekaert et al., 2006).

EARLY IMPACT IN THE UNITED KINGDOM

Small, seemingly unimportant events often have enormous, unlooked-for consequences. When a young Ian Christie settled into his seat in an off-Broadway theatre during the spring of 1968, he was hardly likely to have thought that the clandestine tape-recording he made of the play would spark a virtual revolution in drug treatment across Europe. The previous year, Dr. Christie had taken up his first consultancy post at St. James' Hospital in Portsmouth, United Kingdom. As the new boy, he was given the least attractive job in psychiatry at that time—the addiction treatment unit (Christie, personal communication, September 2005). At that time—and for the first time since the publication of the Rolleston Report in 1926—British policy on drug treatment was about to undergo a momentous change, with general practitioners losing the right to treat addiction with drugs such as heroin and cocaine and the power to prescribe such drugs being vested in drug dependency clinics in psychiatric hospitals (Yates, 2002).

Christie recognized that this would dramatically increase referrals to the small unit he had inherited. He saw too that there would be an urgent requirement for new treatments. His arrival in New York had been inspired by a meeting with Griffith Edwards, a founding father of addiction treatment in the United Kingdom. Edwards himself shortly established Featherstone Lodge (later Phoenix House) in London after being inspired on a recent U.S. visit and advised a fact-finding trip to New York, which produced a short list of people and places to visit. The list included Phoenix House and Daytop Lodge where Christie spent an inspirational weekend. And he sat through a play called *The Concept* where the progress of an individual through this new type of community was laid bare in shocking and emotional detail. Speaking of that time, he noted in a recent interview:

> *I am an atheist. Have been since I was 13. But that experience was literally like a religious conversion. At the time, I didn't recognize how powerful it was. But in fact, I came back from America and I was completely manic.*
> (Christie, personal communication, September 2005)

Armed with little more than his tape of the play, his recollections of a weekend spent at Daytop, and a boundless enthusiasm, Christie returned to Portsmouth and established a makeshift TC (Pink Villa Huts, later Alpha House) in the space of two astonishing, whirlwind weeks.

By a strange coincidence, Martien Kooyman, a young Dutch psychiatrist, was invited to see *The Concept* when it toured the Netherlands 2 years later, with a group of Daytop residents as the cast. Like Christie, Kooyman—who had been managing, without much enthusiasm, a methadone-prescribing clinic in Den Haag, the Netherlands—was astonished. Here in that theatre was living proof that, contrary to the mainstream view in European psychiatry—which held addiction to be an incurable relapsing condition—recovery was not only possible, it was emphatically so (Broekaert et al., 2006)!

To understand the extraordinary impact that concept-based TCs have had upon other UK drug treatment modalities, it is important to understand not only the general mood and nature of those other services at the time of their transposition but also the changes that had been seen in the treatment of the mentally ill and the socially dislocated during the previous decades.

In part, of course, the reason lies in the British view of addiction and drug use at that time. Because the focus of British drug policy (and consequently the British drug treatment system) was firmly upon heroin and cocaine, to the almost total exclusion of the more universally popular amphetamines (Spear, 2005; Yates, 1999), and because these drugs, with their associations with jazz music and Hollywood films, were seen as products of a wayward United States, it was perhaps unsurprising that postwar Britain viewed drug addiction as an American disease that would, presumably, respond to American treatment regimes. Of course, this reframing of the drugs experience as the "fault" of the outsider, the stranger, the foreigner, is common to most cultures (Inglis, 1975; Peele & Brodsky, 1975) and goes only part of the way to explaining a phenomenon of which the legacy within the UK drug field remains clearly discernable more than 40 years later.

The groundbreaking work of Maxwell Jones, Tom Main, and others in the development of so-called "democratic" TCs, first at Hollymoor Hospital, Northfield, and later at the Henderson Hospital, have often been described (Broekaert et al., 1996; Kennard, 1983; Kooyman, 2001). However, with one or two exceptions, at least in the United Kingdom, these experiments were kept within the broad tradition of inpatient psychiatric treatment and were largely unknown outside psychiatry.

Nevertheless, these developments were significant elements of broader changes within psychiatric treatment as a whole. For the previous century, psychiatry had been little more than a specialist branch of the criminal justice system, with psychiatrists providing incarceration and basic remedial treatment for the insane (Berridge, 1999). The impact of the work of Freud, Jung, Klein, and others coupled with the availability of new and powerful drugs had led to dramatic changes in postwar psychiatry. While some of these changes were purely about the use of psychoactive drug treatments to facilitate a more humane management of mental illness, others focused upon the "talking therapies" pioneered by Freud and others, including dynamic psychotherapy, psychoanalysis, and group work, while still others, such as the experiments with LSD and psychodrama at Powick Hospital (Sandison, 1997), were a conscious attempt to marry the two emergent traditions.

Foremost amongst this new radical group of doctors and therapists was the Scottish psychiatrist R. D. Laing. Laing had already been acclaimed for his experimental work in Scotland with the establishment of his "rumpus room" in a Glasgow hospital, when in the 1960s, he took the extraordinary step of moving his patients out of the psychiatric hospital altogether and establishing them in an anarchic TC—Kingsley Hall—in the east end of London (Cooper, 1967; Laing, 1994; Laing, Esterton, & Cooper, 1965). Laing and other members of the Philadelphia Association he established influenced, and in turn were influenced by, patient-led movements such as People Not Psychiatry and the emergent Italian movement Psychiatrica Democratica (Basaglia, 1988; Wilkinson & Cox, 1986). These were movements that brought together mental health patients, radical health workers, and social and political activists in a common cause to promote "community healing" outside the established, hospital-based psychiatric traditions.

Outside the confines of psychiatric medicine, there was a long tradition within Western Europe of the use of small, self-governing communities, particularly in the treatment of maladjusted children. Indeed, it is this work, focusing as it did upon therapeutic interventions with a resistant and antisocial group of young people, that offers the most compelling precedent for the American TC model imported into Europe in the early 1970s.

Among the earliest innovators was August Aichhorn, a Viennese schoolteacher in charge of a complex of reformatories for violent young men. His innovative approach in allowing a limited system of self-governance was noted by Freud and was promoted in the United Kingdom by Freud's daughter Anna, who influenced the early work of Maxwell Jones (Mohr, 1966).

Of equal, if not greater, importance was the work of the American innovator, Homer Lane, with his Little Commonwealth in 1913. Lane's approach, much influenced by Steiner, Montesori, Pestalozzi, and others, was a mixture of tough love, including some corporal punishment, extensive self-government, and hard manual labor. Residents were divided into self-regulating "families" and were paid a wage for their work. This wage was pooled and used to clothe and feed the family. Those who idled and thus reduced the family's income were forcefully reprimanded by their peers in family meetings (Bridgeland, 1971).

Of all the inheritors of the Little Commonwealth innovations, the most important was perhaps David Wills. Wills, a former Borstal housemaster, was employed by the Q Camps Committee, later to evolve into the Planned Environment Therapy Trust, to manage a new experiment with delinquent youths, called the Hawkspur Experiment. Wills, who freely acknowledged his debt, drew heavily upon the work of Lane. The Hawkspur Camp was founded in 1936 with staff and residents living in tents and building their own accommodation. Much of the ethos of the camp was draw from the open-air school movement, but the tough love regime and the self-governing economy were pure Lane (Wills, 1967).

The work of these early innovators was replicated in work with maladjusted children across Europe, although the influence of this pioneering work upon the emergent democratic TC movement is rarely acknowledged. What does seem likely is that this tradition of confrontative group work and self-governance with young delinquents facilitated the establishment of the early addiction TCs, as they began to be imported into Europe in the early 1970s, and ensured that these apparently new ideas were accepted more readily than might otherwise have been the case.

Whatever the reasons, these new TCs soon began to exert an influence upon the field of drug treatment in the United Kingdom, which greatly outstripped their actual practical involvement in the field. By the mid-1970s, concept-based TCs accounted for almost half of the residential rehabilitation beds in the United Kingdom (Yates, 1981). Although this is an impressive "territorial" claim, in terms of numbers of drug users presenting for treatment, TCs were actually a relatively small player. However, their influence was felt throughout the treatment field.

By the mid-1970s, medical staff working in drug dependency units was beginning to incorporate some of the techniques of TCs into the clinical setting. The aim was to provide a more therapeutic regime than the sterile interaction that had developed, largely dominated by staff–patient manipulation around dosage and type of substitute prescription (Mitcheson, 1994). Nonresidential treatment services too were influenced by the TCs, with some developing preentry "induction programs" (Strang & Yates, 1982; Yates, 1979), while others began to undertake group work modeled upon that found in TCs. Similarly, existing residential services were keen to adopt some TC practices, and a number of Christian-based houses began to develop a more hard-edged, confrontative approach to the interactions between residents and staff (Wilson, 1978).

COMMUNITY AS METHOD

At the heart of the TC modality lies the careful balancing of two complementary but polar-opposite elements. Firstly, the TC is characterized by its use of the community itself in creating a day-to-day environment that is designed to aid recovery and learning. De Leon (1997) notes:

> *What distinguishes the TC from other treatment approaches and other communities is the purposive use of the peer community to facilitate social and psychological change in individuals.* (p. 5)

Thus, the daily routine and structure is manipulated to ensure that each member of the community is presented with appropriate and relevant challenges and rewards. A therapeutic environment is not necessarily the same as a supportive one, although challenges must be set in a community within which each individual feels safe and cared for.

Secondly, the rigidity and daily pressure of the work routine is counterbalanced by the use of groups where the hierarchy is abandoned and the rules and ideology can be challenged. This encounter or resolution group system provides the safety valve to the "pressure cooker" of "being on the floor."

This careful juxtapositioning of two opposing elements is at the core of the early success of TCs. Indeed, this balance between a retaining and supportive structure and the provision of a safe haven within which to explore and share experiences of personal vulnerability are seen as central to recovery-oriented interventions in general (Best et al., 2010; Jason, Ferrari, Davis, & Olson, 2006; White, 2008). Subsequent developments in the United Kingdom and elsewhere that have seen the increasing professionalization of the staffing of TCs, while welcome in many respects, has in some cases undermined this delicate balance and damaged the fidelity of the model (De Leon, 2010). Many professional employees entering TCs from other areas of clinical work during that time assumed that individual counseling and group work were the therapeutic inputs, with working "on the floor" merely occupying the spaces in between. This view effectively misses the point. The central tenet of the TC is that it is the day-to-day environment that constitutes the therapeutic input. Formal interventions such as groups merely allow release, understanding, and goal setting.

Thus, creating a working environment that is pressurized, rigorous, and often stressful is the priority and needs to be recognized as the crucial element in the process. The emphasis on individual treatment planning is helpful but needs to be set within the TC context. TCs work by harnessing the power and energy of the group, both staff and residents, and there is a danger that this process can be partially undermined by too great a reliance on individual work. There is good evidence to support the use of interventions such as motivational interviewing, relapse prevention, mindfulness, and other similar interventions that have been embraced by TCs in recent years. However, it should be borne in mind that these are enhancements and not a substitute for the primary TC treatment approach: community as method (De Leon, 2010).

TCs occupy a middle ground between mutual-aid fellowships and mainstream "clinical" treatment. The peer-support and role-modeling elements of mutual-aid fellowships are central to the TC process. The reward and punishment aspects of the resident hierarchy are in many ways similar to—and used in similar ways to—the 12 steps. The differences in the TC model are the intensity of the intervention and the use of challenge and confrontation to point out unacceptable behavior and attitudes. De Leon (2010) and others (Jason et al., 2006; McKeganey, Bloor, Robertson, Neale, & MacDougall, 2006) have argued that some drug users with severe dependence problems will require the intensity of a residentially based intervention. While the use of confrontation has been questioned by White and Miller (2007), De Leon (2000) has argued that it is central to the recovery process, and Jason and colleagues, reporting on a 15-year study of the Oxford House movement, reported that sober-house residents were broadly positive about confrontation and challenge and saw it as an important resource in maintaining their recovery.

TCs have often been criticized for a perceived high dropout rate, particularly within the first months of treatment. However, this is not a problem particular to TCs. Morris and Schultz (1992), in a review of the evidence on treatment retention and compliance appertaining to a range of disorders requiring long-term interventions (including diabetes, hypertension, asthma, etc.), estimated treatment retention at approximately 50%, and various authors (McLellan, Lewis, O'Brien, & Kleber, 2000; O'Brien & McLellan, 1996; White, 2008) have argued that substance use disorders not only require similarly long-term focused treatment, but suffer from similar dropout rates.

Although retention in substitute prescribing treatment is somewhat superior to other addiction treatment modalities in this respect, it is by no means immune to this problem. Simpson, Joe, and Rowan-Szal (1997), in a study involving three methadone treatment programs in Texas, found that two thirds had dropped out within the first 12 months, with one third dropping out in the first 12 weeks. In Italy, D'Ippoliti, Davoli, Perucci, Pasqualini, and Bargagli (1998) surveyed 1,503 heroin addicts entering either methadone maintenance therapy (MMT) or a naltrexone detoxification with a community-based (ambulatory) program of group work and drug counseling. At the end of 12 months, 60% of the MMT clients had dropped out, while in the detoxification group, more than 80% had left treatment.

In various studies of retention in TCs, Lewis and Ross (1994) have noted that the dropout rates differ very little from other addiction treatment modalities. They argue that the bulk of dropouts occur within the first 12 weeks of treatment, with retention rates ranging from 60% to 70% and with a significant reduction in dropout thereafter. Ravndal and Vaglum (1994), in an

18-month study of a TC in Norway, found a retention rate of 25%. Broadly similar rates were reported by De Leon (1991), although De Leon notes that, at that time, retention rates had been improving in TCs throughout the 1980s.

While there has been a great deal of progress regarding the evidence base for various types of addiction treatment intervention, the field remains characterized perhaps more by what we do *not* know than what we *do*. More succinctly, most of the evidence indicates that treatment works, but very little is known about how it works or who it works best for. It is perhaps, therefore, not entirely surprising that many treatment plan decisions are, in practice, based more upon individual beliefs and assumptions than upon any scientific evidence.

Traditionally, residential rehabilitation in general, and TCs in particular, have been seen as effective but expensive interventions, suitable only for a minority of clients whose failure to comply with the requirements of other treatments deemed less expensive warrants the additional expense. As a result, TCs are generally found to cater to a significantly more damaged group of clients (De Leon, Melnick, & Cleland, 2008; Gossop, Marsden, Stewart, & Treacy, 2002; Holt, Ritter, Swann, & Pahoki, 2002; Yates, 2008) than corresponding populations in nonresidential treatment modalities. They have higher levels of mental ill health (Yates, 2008), use a wider range of substances with more frequency (Pitts & Yates, 2010; Yates 2008), and are more persistent users of a wide range of treatment and welfare services (De Leon et al., 2008; Gossop et al., 2002). While these findings are not particularly surprising, it is noticeable that such significant sample differences, with all the attendant implications for prognosis, are largely ignored in various comparative outcome and/or cost-based studies.

THE FALL AND RISE AGAIN OF TCS IN THE UNITED KINGDOM

Despite their early promise and radical approach, TCs in the United Kingdom were slow to adapt to the changing demography as the number of drug users began to spiral at the end of the 1970s (Yates, 1992). With the escalation in drug users came an expansion in drug treatment services, and TCs struggled to make their voice heard in what was now a substantial treatment field dominated by community-based services. This changing emphasis toward outpatient or ambulatory treatments echoed wider developments in UK psychiatry and social welfare. Increasingly, throughout the 1980s, the trend was away from large inpatient psychiatric hospitals and toward a range of treatments in the community. These changes were also accompanied by changes in the care of the elderly and of difficult-to-manage young people and ultimately resulted in the Care in the Community Act of 1990, which established an internal market in public health and further reinforced the "community good–residential bad" message (Yates, 2002, 2003).

Furthermore, increasing alarm at the spread of HIV/AIDS ensured that after less than a decade in the wings, medicine returned to center stage. Almost overnight, the priority client changed from the drug user who wanted to stop using to the one who did not and who therefore presented the greatest risk for the spread of the virus. Effectively, the new political imperative was infection control—now newly labeled as harm reduction—and not recovery. TCs, the arch proponents of recovery, found themselves on the margins of the debate without making any conscious movement. This increasing marginalization was reinforced by changes in the UK public funding of care and resulted in a reallocation of resources to local authorities. This left TCs—which in the United Kingdom had traditionally served a geographically diverse population—negotiating per-capita funding with a large number of local authorities who were only too aware that the purse was limited and that other, more "worthy" causes needed to be funded from within the same allocation. As a result, most TCs in the United Kingdom found themselves under pressure to shorten program lengths, abandon practices with which some funders were uncomfortable, and ensure a higher ratio of "professional" staff. Ironically, as the UK TC movement began to accommodate changes for reasons of survival, they began to lose those distinctive elements that made them a valued contributor to the treatment panoply.

Paradoxically, during the same period, TCs began to be explored by treatment planners within the UK prison system. There is extremely good evidence for TC interventions in custodial institutions (Inciardi, Martin, & Butzin, 2004; Inciardi, Martin, Butzin, Hooper, & Harrison, 1997; Wexler et al., 1997; Wexler, Melnick, Lowe, & Peters, 1999), as there is for the effectiveness of TCs with particularly damaged, dually diagnosed clients (Sacks, De Leon, McKendrick, Brown, & Sacks, 2003; Sacks, Sacks, De Leon, Bernhardt, Staines, 1997; Sacks, Sacks, McKendrick, Banks, & Stommel, 2004).

Clearly, the future for the TC now lies in niche marketing of a kind already beginning to be apparent in some areas. To ensure continued existence and integrity, TCs will in the future, need to target those areas where they can make the most impact and achieve the most good. This means designing modified TCs for particularly vulnerable populations such as the homeless and those with coexisting disorders and establishing TCs in areas where they are likely to attract a higher proportion of their traditional client group, such as in prisons and detention centers. It also means TCs working to reposition themselves as a "senior partner" in the growing UK recovery movement.

The past 5 years in the United Kingdom have seen a resurgence of interest in recovery as a central focus of addiction interventions. In part, this has grown out of a sense of dissatisfaction among the media, policymakers, and service planners with the limited goals of current mainstream addiction treatments. This was perhaps best exemplified by the public debate that followed the BBC's challenging of the National Treatment Agency's annual report in 2007, which appeared to show that only 3% of the treatment population were leaving treatment drug free (Ashton, 2008). In part also though, this passion for recovery appears to have been grounded in a very grassroots revolution, led by service users themselves expressing their disenchantment with a treatment regime that appeared to place a higher priority upon infection control and reductions in offending than on their aspirations to achieve an abstinence-based recovery. This has resulted in the emergence of a number of peer-support initiatives, based loosely upon 12-step principles but espousing a far more muscular approach than that practiced by the traditional mutual-aid fellowships (Gilman & Yates, 2010).

Sociologically, what is fascinating about these recent developments is their startling similarity to the emergence of TCs in the United Kingdom in the early 1970s. Once again, recovery-oriented services are being demanded by a largely service-user led group, joined by practitioners and academics who feel that services can—and should—do more than simply manage and contain the drug-misuse phenomenon. Once again, the movement at its core appears to be profoundly "antitreatment," because "treatment" has increasingly come to be seen as an agent of repression seeking to undermine individual recovery in the service of broader social imperatives. Once again, this is happening at a time when belief in recovery within mainstream treatment services is at an extremely low ebb (Yates, McIvor, Eley, Malloch, & Barnsdale, 2005). Back then, the newly emergent TCs were seen as dangerously close to the fashion for hippy communes and thus dangerously leftwing. Now, this new recovery movement tends to be characterized as a rightwing, outdated, and impractical crusade based more upon faith than science. In both versions, the distortion is aimed at discrediting an aspiration that is seen by mainstream treatment as hopelessly idealistic.

What is clearly required now is for the TC movement and other long-time proponents of abstinence-based recovery to join together with the new recovery movements to reassert the evidence base for recovery. Half a century of field-based outcome studies have shown that recovery through TCs and other peer-support-based interventions is not only possible but scientifically proven (Best et al., 2010; De Leon, 2010; White, 2008).

As long as the recovery movement continues to be distracted by the (already answered) question of *if* such interventions work, the questions of *how* they work and who they work best for will remain unanswered.

REFERENCES

Ashton, M. (2008, December/January). The new abstentionists. *Druglink* (Special Insert). Retrieved from http://www.drugscope.org.uk/Resources/Drugscope/Documents/PDF/Good%20Practice/Ashton_M_30.pdf

Basaglia, F. (1988). Italian psychiatric reform as a reflection of society. In S. Ryan & M. Giannichedda (Eds.), *Psychiatry in transition: The British and Italian experiences* (pp. 141–157). London, United Kingdom: Pluto Press.

Bassin, A. (1978). *The miracle of the TC: From birth to postpartum insanity to full recovery.* Paper presented at the second World Conference of Therapeutic Communities, McGill University, Montreal, Quebec, Canada.

Berridge, V. (1999). *Opium and the people: Opiate use and drug control policy in nineteenth- and early twentieth-century England.* London, United Kingdom: Free Association Books.

Best, D. (2010). Mapping routes to recovery: The role of recovery groups and communities. In R. Yates & M. Malloch (Eds.), *Tackling addiction: Pathways to recovery* (pp. 32–43). London, United Kingdom: Jessica Kingsley.

Best, D., Harris, J., & Strang, J. (2000). The NHS AA/NA: NHS attitudes to 12-step help. *Addiction Today, 11*(65), 17–19.

Best, D., Rome, A., Hanning, K., White, W., Gossop, M., Taylor, A., & Perkins, A. (2010). *Research for recovery: A review of the drugs evidence base.* Edinburgh, Scotland: Scottish Government Social Research.

Bridgeland, M. (1971). *Pioneer work with maladjusted children.* London, United Kingdom: Staples.

Broekaert, E., Bracke, R., Calle, D., Cogo, A., Van Der Straten, G., & Bradt, H. (1996). *De nieuwe therapeutische gemeenschap* [The new therapeutic communities]. Leuven, Belgium: Garant.

Broekaert, E., Vandervelde, S., Soyez, V., Yates, R., & Slater, A. (2006). The third generation of therapeutic communities: The early development of the TC for addiction in Europe. *European Addiction Research, 12*(1), 2–11.

Clarke, L. (2003). *The time of the therapeutic communities: People, places, and events.* London, United Kingdom: Jessica Kingsley.

Cooper, D. (1967). *Psychiatry and antipsychiatry.* London, United Kingdom: Tavistock.

De Leon, G. (1991). Retention in drug-free therapeutic communities. In R. W. Pickens, C. G. Leukefeld, & C. R. Schuster (Eds.), *Improving drug treatment* (NIDA Research Monograph 106). Rockville, MD: National Institute on Drug Abuse.

De Leon, G. (Ed.). (1997). *Community as method: Therapeutic communities for special populations and special settings.* Westport, CT: Praeger.

De Leon, G. (2000). *The therapeutic community: Theory, model, and method.* New York, NY: Springer.

De Leon, G. (2010). Is the therapeutic community an evidence-based treatment? What the evidence says. *International Journal of Therapeutic Communities, 31*(2), 104–128.

De Leon, G., Melnick, G., & Cleland, C. (2008). Client matching: A severity–treatment intensity paradigm. *Journal of Addictive Diseases, 27*(3), 99–113.

D'Ippoliti, D., Davoli, M., Perucci, C. A., Pasqualini, F., & Bargagli, A. M. (1998). Retention in treatment of heroin users in Italy: The role of treatment type and of methadone maintenance dosage. *Drug & Alcohol Dependence, 52*, 167–171.

Dole, V. P., & Nyswander, M. (1965). A medical treatment for diacetylmorphine (heroin) addiction: A clinical trial with methadone hydrochloride. *Journal of the American Medical Association, 193*, 646–650.

Gilman, M., & Yates, R. (2010). NW ROIS: Recovery-oriented integrated systems in North West England. In R. Yates & M. Malloch (Eds.), *Tackling addiction: Pathways to recovery* (pp. 84–95). London, United Kingdom: Jessica Kingsley.

Gossop, M., Marsden, J., Stewart, D., & Treacy, S. (2002). Change and stability of change after treatment of drug misuse: 2-year outcomes from the National Treatment Outcome Research Study (UK). *Addictive Behaviors, 27*, 155–166.

Holt, T., Ritter, A., Swann, A., & Pahoki, S. (2002). *Australian treatment outcome survey (ATOS)*. Fitzroy, Victoria, Australia: Turning Point Alcohol & Drug Center.

Inciardi, J., Martin, S., & Butzin, C. (2004). Five-year outcomes of therapeutic community treatment of drug-involved offenders after release from prison. *Crime & Delinquency, 50*(1), 88–107.

Inciardi, J. A., Martin, S. S., Butzin, C. A., Hooper, R. M., & Harrison, L. D. (1997). An effective model of prison-based treatment for drug-involved offenders. *Journal of Drug Issues, 27*(2), 261–278.

Inglis, B. (1975). *The forbidden game: A social history of drugs*. London, United Kingdom: Hodder & Stoughton.

Jason, L. A., Ferrari, J. R., Davis, M. I., & Olson, B. D. (Eds.). (2006). *Creating communities for addiction recovery: The Oxford House model*. Binghamton, NY: Haworth.

Kennard, D. (1983). *An introduction to therapeutic communities*. London, United Kingdom: Routledge & Kegan Paul.

Kooyman, M. (1992). *The therapeutic community for addicts: Intimacy, parent involvement, and treatment outcome*. Lisse, The Netherlands: Swets & Zeitlinger.

Kooyman, M. (2001). The history of therapeutic communities: A view from Europe. In B. Rawlings & R. Yates (Eds.), *Therapeutic communities for the treatment of drug users* (pp. 110–156). London, United Kingdom: Jessica Kingsley Publishers.

Laing, A. (1994). *R. D. Laing: A life*. London, United Kingdom: Harper Collins.

Laing, R., Esterton, A., & Cooper, D. (1965). Results of family-oriented therapy with hospitalized schizophrenics. *British Medical Journal, 2*, 1462–1465.

Lewis, B. F., & Ross, R. (1994). Retention in therapeutic communities: Challenges for the nineties. In F. M. Timms, G. De Leon, & N. Jainchill (Eds.), *Therapeutic community: Advances in research and application* (NIDA Research Monograph Series 144; pp. 99–116). Rockville, MD: NIDA.

Louria, D. B. (1968). *The drug scene*. New York, NY: McGraw-Hill Book Company.

McKeganey, N. P., Bloor, M. J., Robertson, M., Neale, J., & MacDougall, J. (2006). Abstinence and drug abuse treatment: Results from the Drug Outcome Research in Scotland Study. *Drugs: Education, Prevention, and Policy, 13*(6), 537–550.

McLellan, A. T., Lewis, D. C., O'Brien, C. P., & Kleber, H. D. (2000). Drug dependence, a chronic medical illness: Implications for treatment, insurance, and outcomes evaluation. *Journal of the American Medical Association, 284*(13), 1719–1720.

Mitcheson, M. (1994). Drug clinics in the 1970s. In J. Strang & M. Gossop (Eds.), *Heroin addiction and drug policy: The British system* (pp. 178–191). Oxford, United Kingdom: Oxford University Press.

Mohr, G. (1966). August Aichhorn. In F. Alexander, S. Einstein, & M. Grotjahn (Eds.), *Psychoanalytic pioneers*. New York, NY: Basic Books.

Morris, L., & Schultz, R. (1992). Patient compliance: An overview. *Journal of Clinical Pharmacy and Therapeutics, 17*(5), 283–295.

O'Brien, C. P., & McLellan, A. T. (1996). Myths about the treatment of addiction. *The Lancet, 347*(8996), 237–240.

Peele, S., & Brodsky, A. (1975). *Love and addiction*. New York, NY: Taplinger.

Pitts, J., & Yates, R. (2010). Cost benefits of therapeutic community programming: Results of a self-funded survey. *International Journal of Therapeutic Communities, 31*, 129–144.

Ravndal, E. (2003). Research in the concept-based therapeutic community—its importance to European treatment research in the drug field. *International Journal of Social Welfare, 12*, 229–238.

Ravndal, E., & Vaglum, P. (1994). Self-reported depression as a predictor of dropout in a hierarchical therapeutic community. *Journal of Substance Abuse Treatment, 11*, 471–479.

Rawlings, B., & Yates, R. (2001). Fallen angel: An introduction. In B. Rawlings & R. Yates (Eds.), *Therapeutic communities for the treatment of drug users* (pp. 6–46). London, United Kingdom: Jessica Kingsley.

Robins, L., & Murphy, G. (1967). Drug use in a normal population of young negro men. *American Journal of Public Health, 57*, 1580–1586.

Roman, P. M., Johnson, J. A., Ducharme, L., Knudsen, H., & Meredith, P. H. (2005). *Summary report: A national sample of therapeutic communities* (Report No. 9). Athens, GA: National Treatment Center, University of Georgia.

Sacks, S., De Leon, G., McKendrick, K., Brown, B., & Sacks, J. Y. (2003). TC-oriented supported housing for homeless MICAs. *Journal of Psychoactive Drugs, 35*(3), 355–366.

Sacks, S., Sacks, J. Y., De Leon, G., Bernhardt, A. I., & Staines, G. L. (1997). Modified therapeutic community for mentally ill chemical 'abusers': Background, influences, program description, preliminary findings. *Substance Use and Misuse, 32*(9), 1217–1259.

Sacks, S., Sacks, J. Y., McKendrick, K., Banks, S., & Stommel, J. (2004). Modified TC for MICA offenders: Crime outcomes. *Behavioral Sciences and the Law, 22*, 477–501.

Sandison, R. (1997). LSD therapy: A retrospective. In A. Melechi (Ed.), *Psychedelia Britannica: Hallucinogenic drugs in Britain*. London, United Kingdom: Turnaround.

Simpson, D. D., Joe G. W., & Rowan-Szal, G. (1997). Drug abuse treatment retention and process effects on follow-up outcomes. *Drug and Alcohol Dependence, 47*, 227–235.

Spear, H. B. (2005). The early years of Britain's drug situation in practice: Up to the 1960s. In J. Strang & M. Gossop (Eds.), *Heroin addiction and drug policy: The British System* (Vol. 1, pp. 17–42). Oxford, United Kingdom: Oxford University Press.

Strang, J., & Yates, R. (1982). *Involuntary treatment and addiction*. Strasbourg, France: Council of Europe (Pompidou Group).

Vaillant, G. (1966). A 12-year follow-up study of New York narcotic addicts. *American Journal of Psychiatry, 122,* 727–735.

Vandevelde, S. (1999). *Maxwell Jones and his work in the therapeutic community.* Unpublished doctoral dissertation, Universiteit Ghent. Retrieved from http://www.drugslibrary.stir.ac.uk/documents/vandevelde1999.pdf

Wexler, H. K., Melnick, G., Lowe, L., & Peters, J. (1999). Three-year reincarceration outcomes for Amity in-prison therapeutic community and aftercare in California. *Prison Journal, 79*(3), 312–336.

White, W. (2000). The history of recovered people as wounded healers: From Native America to the rise of the modern alcoholism movement. *Alcoholism Treatment Quarterly, 18,* 1–23.

White, W. (2008). *Recovery management and recovery-oriented systems of care: Scientific rationale and promising practices.* Philadelphia, PA: North East Addiction Technology Transfer Centre/Great Lakes Addiction Technology Transfer Centre/Philadelphia Department of Behavioral Health & Mental Retardation Services.

White, W., & Miller, W. (2007). The use of confrontation in addiction treatment: History, science, and time for change. *Counselor, 8*(4), 12–30.

Wilkinson, K., & Cox, A. (1986). Principles into practice: A developmental study of a community mental health service. Manchester, United Kingdom: Youth Development Trust.

Wills, D. (1967). The Hawkspur Experiment. London, United Kingdom: Allen & Unwin.

Wilson, F. W. (1978). Spiritual therapy in the therapeutic community. In P. Vamos, & D. Brown (Ed.), *Proceedings of the Second World Conference of Therapeutic Communities: The Addiction Therapist, Special Edition, 4,* 204–205.

Winick, C. (1962). Maturing out of narcotic addiction. *United Nations Bulletin on Narcotics, 14*(1), 1–7.

Yablonsky, L. (1965). *Synanon: The tunnel back.* New York, NY: Macmillan.

Yates, R. (1979). An experiment in multifacility addiction. In P. Vamos & D. Brown (Eds.), *Proceedings of the Second World Conference of Therapeutic Communities: The Addiction Therapist, Special Edition, 3,* 25–30.

Yates, R. (1981). *Out from the shadows.* London, United Kingdom: National Association for the Care and Resettlement of Offenders.

Yates, R. (1992). *If it weren't for the alligators: A history of drugs, music, & popular culture in Manchester.* Manchester, United Kingdom: Lifeline Project.

Yates, R. (1999). Only available in black: The limiting of addiction services in the 20th century. In *Uteseksjonen 30 Ar Pa Gata, November 1999* (pp. 2–11). Oslo, Norway: Uteseksjonen. http://www.drugslibrary.stir.ac.uk/documents/black.pdf

Yates, R. (2002). A brief history of British drug policy, 1950–2001. *Drugs, Education, Prevention, and Policy, 9,* 113–124.

Yates, R. (2003). A brief moment of glory: The impact of the therapeutic community movement on drug treatment systems in the UK. *International Journal of Social Welfare, 12*(3), 239–243.

Yates, R. (2008). Different strokes for different folks: Results of a small study comparing characteristics of a therapeutic community population with a community drug project population. *International Journal of Therapeutic Communities*, *29*(1), 44–56.

Yates, R., & Malloch, M. (2010). The road less traveled? A short history of addiction recovery. In R. Yates & M. Malloch (Eds.), *Tackling addiction: Pathways to recovery* (pp. 15–31). London, United Kingdom: Jessica Kingsley.

Yates, R., McIvor, G., Eley, S., Malloch, M., & Barnsdale, L. (2005, November). Coercion in drug treatment: The impact on motivation, aspiration, and outcome. In M. Pedersen, V. Segraeus, & M. Hellman (Eds.), *Evidence-based practice—Challenges in substance abuse treatment: Proceedings of the 7th International Symposium on Substance Treatment* (pp. 159–170). Helsinki, Norway: Nordic Council for Alcohol and Drug Research/University of Aarhus/European Working Group on Drugs Oriented Research/European Federation of Therapeutic Communities.

The Challenge of Developing and Sustaining a Recovery Group in Glasgow: Calton Athletic Recovery Group

MARGARET S. MALLOCH

Scottish Centre for Crime and Justice Research, University of Stirling, Stirling, United Kingdom

This article will consider how Calton Athletic Recovery Group (CARG) defines and supports recovery and will examine the challenges inherent in setting up and sustaining a project that has a primary aim to "bring recovery into the community." Based in the East end of Glasgow, the project was set up in 1985 as a football team and social group aimed at supporting and sustaining recovery from drug and alcohol problems. In the 25 years that CARG has been in existence, it has experienced highs and lows in terms of funding, resources, and wider support. The issues of sustainability and community identity are considered as experienced by the members of CARG.

INTRODUCTION

In 2008, the same year that the Scottish Government launched the new drug policy *The Road to Recovery*, I was conducting a small research project (supported by the Carnegie Trust) to examine the role of "grassroots" community-based organizations and the impact they have on personal and community processes of recovery. As part of this project, I contacted Calton Athletic Recovery Group (CARG), a group that was founded in 1985 as a football team and social club run by, and for, recovering drug addicts.[1] CARG was

The author wishes to thank David Bryce and members of the Calton Athletic Recovery Group; and David Best and the anonymous referees for their helpful comments on an earlier version of this paper.

based in Calton, a district in the East end of Glasgow—an area characterized by high rates of social deprivation and problem drug use.[2]

During the 1980s and 1990s, the success of CARG captured the imagination of many and led to increased publicity for the group. The BBC drama *Alive and Kicking* (1991) was based on the CARG concept, and the involvement of the group in the production of *Trainspotting* (1996) further increased their public profile. However, funding difficulties and the restructuring of drug services in Glasgow led to ongoing concerns over the future of CARG. In the wake of newspaper reports that CARG faced imminent closure (Morgan, 1992) or had indeed closed (Nutt, 2000), I was keen to find out if CARG was still "alive and kicking."

Contact with CARG's founder and director, David Bryce, proved that while CARG may have slipped from wider public awareness, the group was very much alive and active in 2008 and continuing to work steadily with men.[3] The group did not have any form of funding; there were no paid workers or administrative support, and the group was essentially self-supporting. However, men continued to access the service through established group members, and examples of healthy and sustained recovery were evident. More than just a "sports" or a "drugs" project, CARG continued to operate as a community project aimed at changing lives through recovery.

This article considers the development of CARG and what "recovery" means for the group, identifies strengths and challenges, and indicates benefits that CARG has made in the lives of those who engaged with the provisions available. Clearly, not everyone who has contact with CARG is able or willing to adhere to the requirements of attendance (i.e., remaining drug and alcohol free), and as with all services in this field, some individuals will be limited in their ability to sustain recovery at a particular point in time. However, as the article illustrates, it has succeeded in making significant changes in the lives of those who have participated. By encouraging and supporting recovery in the men who take part, the consequences go beyond, to families and communities in which the men live and work.[4]

The example of CARG highlights a number of pertinent issues that will be considered. Like other community-based support groups, it provides an example of a path to recovery essentially beyond the statutory sector; and this disengagement with "official" services can often mean that access to funds is curtailed. While *The Road to Recovery* is an inclusive approach to responding to drug problems (and parallels a focus on recovery in the United States), the challenges of bringing all relevant agencies together is not without difficulty. This involves drawing together organizations with a fundamentally different way of defining the drug problem in Scotland; subsequently, the ideological implications arising from these definitions result in different views of an appropriate response.[5] Although the spirit of Scotland's drug policy is inclusive and creates opportunities for different definitions of "recovery" and different means of accessing it, in practice, this is a complex and potentially challenging task (Best et al., 2008). Establishing criteria for funding requires that mechanisms of accountability through monitoring and evaluation are in place and may be better established where agencies are aligned with statutory services, or indeed, have developed with these processes embedded in service design. While recovery may be a fledgling concept in policy priorities, organizations such as CARG that have consistently emphasized recovery as their fundamental basis can still experience difficulties in finding acceptance from mainstream services.

BACKGROUND AND DEVELOPMENT OF CARG

CARG developed from the experience of its founder member and current director, David Bryce.[6] Originating from his experience of recovery, CARG was set up to support others to become drug free. A recovery program was established for individuals who wanted to be drug and alcohol free; abstinence was, and remains, a condition of attendance. Attendees receive individual and group counseling and can take part in a range of activities aimed at character building. Sport and fitness activities are part of a package of self-improvement tools, while the influence of peers provides opportunities to change behavior and attitudes. In 1 year, 112 clients completed the program (see CARG Web site, http://www.caltonathletic.com).

Funding (from donations and voluntary sector organizations such as the Robertson Trust, Greater Glasgow Health Board, and Strathclyde Regional Council) provided a range of activities: support to access training and employment, continuous aftercare in the form of evening meetings and weekend activities, a women's service, telephone helpline, and family support. A schools prevention project provided by the CARG Schools Drug Awareness Team was established in 1994 and was made up of drug-free graduates who gave presentations on drug misuse and the effect of this on their lives and the lives of their families (evaluated by McKeganey & McPike, 1997). Awareness raising and training sessions were also provided to agencies and private sector organizations. Fundraising activities provided support for attendance at major football tournaments, a number of which were international.

The development of CARG was characterized by two main features: It was welcomed by those who believed in an abstinence-based approach to the drug problem (and prevention). This led to a significant media interest (the group was involved in advising the makers of *Trainspotting* [1996] in 1995). At the same time, their principled stance brought them into ongoing conflict with other agencies operating in Glasgow, and this resulted in a number of disagreements with funders and service providers (see Bryce & Pia, 2005). While remaining committed to their work with individuals, CARG became increasingly isolated from professional service providers. CARG, although achieving significant publicity and renown, in effect seemed to be caught between its primary focus of attaining and sustaining individual recovery within the local community and attempting to challenge the wider drug treatment community in Scotland at practice and policy levels.

Despite ongoing controversies around service provision and funding issues, the group went from strength to strength during the 1990s. At one point, CARG had three premises in Glasgow from which their services (detoxification support, mentoring, training and employment support, aftercare, dedicated service for women, and the helpline) were provided and from which a range of programs were made available (recovery focused and physical activity based). The demand for their services was evidenced by the number of people who came to CARG looking for help. Although referrals from other agencies were low (most of those attending CARG in 1995 were self-referred), by 1997, the demand for the service was so great that a waiting list was drawn up. To sustain those on the list, a beginner's program was introduced to provide support and retain those in need of the service. Increased funding was secured in subsequent years, and it expanded the number of paid staff and developed prevention work in schools.

By 2000, however, disagreement with funders over the development of the service and restructuring of drug and alcohol services in Glasgow resulted in the depletion and finally the end of CARG's funding from the statutory sector. The group, which still retains an office in the East end of Glasgow supported by members' contributions (although without any staff or administrative support), remains outside the officially recognized network of drug services. The limited resources have raised ongoing concerns about the sustainability of the project and have meant that much focus is required on "keeping things going," while opportunities for expansion and promotion have presented real challenges for CARG. The experience of the group highlights some of the fundamental difficulties in defining and achieving "recovery" through a policy framework approach.

WHAT RECOVERY MEANS TO CARG

CARG employs a specific understanding of what recovery entails. According to David Bryce, it means *"abstinence from drugs and alcohol (...). Recovery means change; rehabilitation; (...) it's not enough to be abstinent, you have to have a willingness to change"* (2010, p. 107). The group's program is loosely based on a 12-step approach,[7] a set of guiding principles outlining a course of action for recovery from addiction. CARG emphasizes the importance of setting out a "program of change" for all participants based on the development and sustenance of honesty, integrity, personal responsibility, responsibilities toward others (family, friends, society), and working to help others with similar problems ("giving something back").[8] However, a key component of the group program is the emphasis given to physical activity as a main focus for change; CARG initially developed this through the establishment of a football team and expanded to include a range of other activities. This approach is seen as an important way of helping individuals transform themselves physically and mentally and develop a sense of camaraderie, and is seen as a means of attracting others to become part of the group. It provides a focus (for achievement) and a productive use of time. Participation in support groups, in combination with other group activities, has been shown to be particularly effective at sustaining abstinence and enhancing health and well-being over time (Humphreys et al., 2004).

A relatively formalized process of progression is in place:

- Assessment

  All potential participants receive an individual assessment (currently undertaken by the director and/or deputy director). They are made aware of the requirements of participation (abstinence from alcohol and drugs), and health and fitness needs are identified. Support will be provided while the individual comes off drink and/or drugs; however, if additional support is required or if the individual does not believe he can meet the requirements of CARG, he will be referred elsewhere.

- Intervention

  Following the initial assessment (individuals will continue to be monitored and supported throughout their involvement), the participant will be linked in with a mentor who will support them on an ongoing and accessible basis. Education about staying sober and drug free in the community will be provided, and the individual will embark on a 3-month structured program. This will involve physical activities (training at the gym, football, and other events), attendance at the weekly recovery group, and ongoing contact with other group members. Individual support will be available from more experienced group members who are able to share their own life experiences with newer men. The structured activities will take place during 3 to 4 days per week, and contact with other group members is expected on a daily basis.

- Aftercare

  After completing the 3-month intensive element of the program, men are expected to remain in contact with their mentor and other group members by involvement in organized activities in addition to attendance at the weekly recovery group; they are supported while their families and relationships are reconciled, and are assisted in finding full-time paid employment, or in developing the skills necessary to achieve this.

While adopting an eclectic approach that has been tried and tested over the years, the basis for CARG's program structure can be linked to a range of therapeutic interventions that have been widely used and accepted in the mental health and substance recovery fields (including 12-step and mutual aid, group psychotherapy and dynamics, and therapeutic community; White & Kurtz, 2005, 2006; Yates & Malloch, 2010). However, the absence of "professional" therapists or counselors contributes to the "down to earth" approach of CARG members, who have developed the program based on their own personal and collective experiences of "what works," and in doing so, they have drawn on interventions acknowledged as "effective" in other arenas.

The combination of individual motivation and group support, along with the support of peers and families, has been noted as particularly beneficial in sustaining recovery (Gyarmathy & Latkin, 2008). The emphasis given to sport and physical activity has also been shown to have important benefits in promoting prevention strategies (Flint, Crawford, Parr, & Powell, 2010) as well as in supporting recovery (Faulkner & Taylor, 2005). Separated, as CARG members currently are, from identified funding streams and the contingent bureaucracies that can be attached has allowed them to develop a program and mode of working relatively unhindered. However, the lack of financial and indeed practical support to develop their work has brought its own challenges. To enhance the sustainability of the organization, CARG has sought to share its experience and to form alliances with organizations with a similar ethos in other parts of Scotland.

Figure 1 highlights the range of services that are made available.

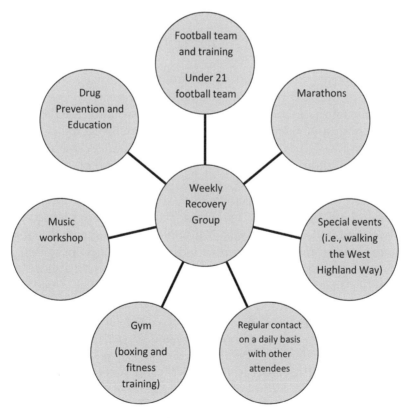

FIGURE 1 Activities

All CARG members are expected to attend the weekly recovery group, which forms the central hub of the program. Other activities are organized through contact established at this meeting and fit in with participants' daily routines (i.e., regular contact with others, attendance at the gym). Some activities are taken up by those with particular interests or enthusiasm to develop specific skills (i.e., music workshop, football team). Other events (participating in marathons, West Highland Way, providing drug prevention and education to other organizations) take place on a regular basis, are open to all, and are instigated and arranged by group members.

The range of activities that group members participate in, as shown above, is significant and revolves around the weekly recovery meeting, which is seen as a crucial part of the service. Members are responsible for providing mutual support to others, although the capacity of CARG to bring in large numbers of new members is limited as most of the men who have attained ongoing recovery move on to full-time employment. Length of recovery is a defining feature of each individual's responsibility for helping newer members. Average attendance at the weekly recovery meeting is 12 to 15 participants. One of the strengths of the group is its ability to attract and sustain young men (in their 20s), who often struggle to engage with other agencies.

METHODOLOGY

As noted previously, this article does not attempt to provide a formal evaluation of CARG; instead, it presents issues and experiences as encountered by the participants in their attempts to develop and sustain CARG as an "effective" recovery group. Background material and archived information were obtained from CARG and from local and national media coverage. Ongoing contact with the group has continued during the course of 2 years.

The views and experiences of CARG members were obtained from attendance at two recovery meetings and from subsequent interviews with 11 men and the CARG director in August 2009.[9] Interviews were recorded, transcribed, and coded for analysis. A number of subsequent meetings took place with CARG's director. The respondents were aged between 23 and 60 years, and length of sobriety ranged from 3 months to more than 30 years, with the majority of respondents (8 of the 11) having stayed drug and alcohol free at CARG for more than 4 years. Six of the respondents were under the age of 33 years. Most, but not all, of the men had been involved with the criminal justice system, and some had served time in prison.

PARTICIPANT VIEWS OF CARG

All of the men who attended the group spoke of the changes that had occurred in their lives since coming to CARG and finding a way to address alcohol and/or drug problems. They talked about the importance of being reunited with their families and of the changes that their recovery had and continued to bring to their relationships. They gave examples of the things they had achieved since coming to CARG—obtaining employment, going to college, staying well—and they talked of the dreams and aspirations they now had for the future. As one respondent commented: "It wasn't that we didn't have ambitions; we were full of them. Drink and drugs got in the way."

Respondents indicated that they had heard of CARG in various ways: through word of mouth, friends and family, at the gym, contact with the football team, or in prison. In recent years, with no dedicated premises for making formal contact, men reported that they would go along to the weekly recovery meeting or to the gym where CARG members have a regular presence to make initial contact with the group. This informal access to CARG, several respondents stated, had enabled them to get the help they needed and provided a way to access help without going through any "official" process to make contact.

At the weekly recovery meeting, the men have an opportunity to meet together, to offer and obtain support from each other, share their experiences, and energize their recovery. While the physical activities were seen as crucial in developing a healthy lifestyle, friendship, and camaraderie, the meetings and ongoing contact among the group were viewed as equally, and in some cases, more, important:

> We are able to be there for each other. It's not just a physical thing, like meeting down the gym; everybody has a phone number, everybody has a contact number. It's a bond between us all.

Respondents described the importance of taking part in the physical activities and the fact that this helped them to prove their capabilities to themselves and others. They also commented that physical exercise was important in managing a "racing mind" or in keeping their thinking straight. One respondent commented:

> It's putting it into action and doing things down the gym. Going out running, that was a main thing as well, doing the runs every Saturday and the Thursdays, it kept us going. It was kind of ... bonding with the boys. We bonded through the gym, through the physical work we did.

At the same time, he notes how the meetings helped too:

> You just ... kind of clear your head. Because it's hard out there, there is a lot of drink, drugs, and there is a lot of temptation, so you need to come here and they say it cleanses you. You get it out, what's been bothering you through the week ...

Another respondent made the same point:

> Definitely, the meetings are a place to empty your head. This is prob-
> ably one of the most important ... for me anyway ... this is the most
> important part of Calton Athletic for me. I love the bonding that we get
> camping; I love the bonding that we get going up hills, doing all the half
> marathons, doing the 10ks; I love the bonding with setting up the mu-
> sic workshop and playing the guitars and the instruments together. But
> this (the recovery meeting) is probably the most important part for me,
> somewhere I can get the madness out of my head and there is somebody
> there to listen, you know?

Making Changes

Much of the strength of CARG comes from its ability to inspire others through
the power of example. One respondent noted that other group members
have lifestyles they can identify with and so will be influenced by them.
Commenting on an older group member who had served a relatively long
prison sentence, he stated:

> From the outside, it sounds silly, but to young guys growing up, that's
> the people we look up to, that's the people you identify with. The gang
> stuff ... that's the lifestyle you always wanted growing up. Now there is
> somebody saying, 'Right, well I've done it and now I've got out of it. I
> am showing you how to get out of it.'

One man commented that his use of drugs stopped him from maturing. He
pointed out:

> Any drug at all that you take stops you from maturing. So my body has
> got older and older and my head has stayed the same age. You get to
> the Calton and your body gets younger and younger and your head gets
> older (laughter). That's the best way I can describe it.

This process of supporting each other and strengthening one's own
recovery by sharing and learning from personal experience is evident in
mutual-aid societies and is considered to be a key element for enhancing
recovery itself. In the process of supporting each other, the bonds of community are created and sustained.

Helping Others

Commitment to helping others is another element of the CARG philosophy,
both in terms of helping each other and helping other people understand

the difficulties that drugs can cause for some individuals. One of the men talked about the importance of the service provided to schools by CARG as he viewed it:

> The school team is by far the best thing that I have ever done because it's about prevention rather than cure; prevention is always better than cure ... I was the supervisor of the school team for over 3 years and I spoke to all the kids and I know the effect and impact it had on them.

Another respondent spoke of the importance of the sense of community that CARG has to offer:

> The first thing they get at Calton Athletic is hope that it can be done. Then they start to get inspired by the people around about them. It's as simple as that. It is a community, it's a sober community, and it works.

The principle of mutual aid is emphasized at CARG, and respondents commented on their responsibility to help others:

> Oh, I come to a meeting every Thursday. Sometimes I feel I don't need a meeting. I always come because there are people here that need to hear what I say and I can always say something that will help other people. Once you get to maybe 2 years, 3 years, it's not about yourself anymore, it's about helping others.

While this commitment is evident in CARG as a community, it has an impact beyond the group; participants are encouraged to develop the same attitude toward others outside the group. This involves (re)establishing and enhancing relationships with family members—parents, children, partners—making a positive contribution in the workplace, and presenting oneself as a "good example" in the community, thereby evidencing the benefits of recovery to others and potentially encouraging others who may be experiencing problems with addiction to come along to CARG.

FUTURE DEVELOPMENT

CARG has the experience and expertise of supporting people into recovery and of sustaining that recovery. Thinking ahead is one of the current challenges for the group, and they are actively seeking funding and the support of other services in the drug and alcohol field. There was an acknowledgement among respondents that although things were working very well for the men who attended CARG, the current set up (i.e., no funding) makes it difficult to support greater numbers of people seeking help.

The way forward is to make it easy for people to get to Calton Athletic; obviously given the number of people who come to the club means that we need resources to deliver the service. If we had the resources, we could reconstruct the services more or less immediately.

CARG members who had been involved as the group expanded and contracted spoke of the expertise that CARG had to offer:

We have still got all the experience to pass on to the younger ones, and that's my philosophy in life. I am just hoping to see the school team getting reestablished again, and it would be good to get the program back onboard again for new people coming. We have got so much to offer people ...

CARG members continue to be active in providing drug information sessions when requested (to schools, football teams), and a number of past graduates have moved on to become drug support workers with other (funded) agencies.

Despite the absence of any support from statutory services, CARG continues to make a major impact on the lives of the men who attend—evidenced by the length of recovery of many and the emphasis on working with others who express a desire to become and remain drug and alcohol free. The emphasis on mutual support and learning from shared experiences is indicative of the recognition by UKDPC (2008, p. 8) that "the development of recovery-oriented services will require a different relationship between service users and professionals and thus there will be many challenges in adopting this approach."

The current Scottish drugs strategy, *Road to Recovery* (Scottish Government, 2008, 2009) is in its 2nd year of operation. The policy emphasizes an eclectic approach to service provision, with recovery identified as a central pillar of the policy; it draws on a range of approaches to encourage individuals to begin their recovery journeys out of addiction. It claims to set out a new vision where all services in the field of drug treatment and rehabilitation are based on the principle of recovery. Recovery is defined in the policy as: "a process through which an individual is enabled to move on from their problem drug use towards a drug-free life and become an active and contributing member of society."

The *Road to Recovery* (Scottish Government, 2008, paragraph 82) sets out the meaning of recovery to the individual, notes that it will mean different things at different points in time, and indicates that recovery goes beyond abstinence (see also Laudet, 2007; White & Kurtz, 2005, 2006). However, it comments:

Above all, people aspiring to milestones in recovery must have the confidence that they can achieve their personal goals (...). Milestones could be as simple as gaining weight, re-establishing relationships with friends, or building self-esteem. What is key is that recovery is sustained.

There is little doubt that CARG supports individuals to achieve these things, to go beyond this, and to continue to support individuals on a long-term basis. It provides an example of what current policy holds up as a successful recovery community. CARG members continue their attempts to obtain support from politicians, policymakers, and charitable funders to access renewed sources of funding and to reestablish their preventative work in schools. The current emphasis on "recovery" clearly fits with the group's philosophy and approach. That they have continued to exist without funding is testament to the group's commitment to provide a service, based on their own experience, to others struggling to address drug and alcohol problems. And although they are currently limited in the extent to which they are embraced by wider community networks, the group effectively provides an active "community of recovery" to the participants (White & Kurtz, 2006) and their families. Indeed, they appear to provide an environment where "recovery capital" (Cloud & Granfield, 2008; White & Kurtz, 2005) can be enhanced significantly. This manifests itself in the local community by strengthening the wider benefits that arise from individuals who are able to make a substantial contribution to society through taking responsibility for their lives, employment, and families, and who are keen to "give something back" to their community.

The historical split between abstinence and harm-reduction approaches has been acknowledged as divisive, and emphasis has been given to the need for a broad range of "pathways to recovery" (Scottish Advisory Committee on Drug Misuse, 2008; UKDPC, 2008), although caution is expressed by Best et al. (2008) in suggesting that all potential pathways are equal in the "recovery" they can realistically attain. CARG can usefully offer its particular approach (abstinence based) for those who are willing to take this path. However, the difficulties facing a group such as CARG remain. Funders require built-in processes of monitoring and evaluation to evidence "effectiveness" in services; and "outcomes" are not universally agreed (Laudet, 2007). Although CARG is able to evidence this through the individual experiences of members who are in recovery as a direct result of their involvement with the group, it recognizes the need to implement processes of accountability. However, without any administrative support, this is a current challenge for the group (i.e., there is no funding to support data collection or monitoring systems; without data collection or monitoring systems, there is no tangible way of obtaining funding). Another challenge is the difficult one that arises when small but successful organizations become co-opted into funding streams. They can lose their autonomy and drive as a result of the requirements placed upon them by funders.[10]

The experiences of CARG serve to highlight the important provision they can continue to make in supporting recovery as an experience, at the same time illustrating the challenges for a recovery-based policy agenda that attempts to support recovery as a measurable entity.

There are a number of wider recovery lessons that can be learned from the experience of CARG. The group illustrates the immense amount that can be achieved by nonprofessionals who are working together (with and without funding) and who are united by a shared experience and coherent focus. The important role of one or two determined individuals in developing and sustaining this focus is also evident. The difficulties of transferring this "determination" to a professional, statutory way of working can present real challenges in terms of philosophy and practice, highlighting the importance of recognizing different pathways to recovery and ensuring that groups such as CARG are acknowledged for the impact they are able to make in sustaining recovery.

NOTES

1. This information on which this article is based was collated as part of a larger study and does not attempt to provide an "evaluation" of the project.

2. The Calton area of Glasgow has the lowest average male life expectancy in Scotland (at 53.9 years). This is considerably lower than life expectancy in (for example) Iraq (67.49 years) and the Gaza Strip (70.5 years; General Register Office for Scotland, 2010).

3. While CARG has provided a service for women in the past, it now focuses solely on working with men.

4. The article does not present views from the wider community; this important insight could usefully be obtained for the future.

5. There have been ongoing debates (see, for example, the New Abstentionists debate; Best, Loaring, Ghufran, & Day, 2008; Scotland's Future's Forum, 2008; UK Drug Policy Commission [UKDPC], 2008)

6. See David's book *Alive and Kicking*, with Simon Pia (2005), for a more detailed account.

7. Originally proposed by Alcoholics Anonymous (AA) as a method of recovery from alcoholism, the 12 steps were first published in the book, *Alcoholics Anonymous*, in 1939. Twelve-step programs have received particular attention from professionals advocating the importance of "recovery" as a priority for drug treatment services.

8. The importance of individuals in recovery helping others to recover is now acknowledged as crucial in sustaining long-term recovery (see White & Kurtz, 2006). This recognition has informed the current Scottish Drugs Strategy.

9. It was not possible to obtain quantitative data about the previous or current operation of the group. However, given the importance of statistical data to support the effective operation of organizations in general (i.e., outputs, outcomes), this is an area that CARG is currently attempting to develop.

10. This concern led to the development of AA as a completely self-financing organization (see Kurtz, 1979). Humphreys et al. (2004, p. 156) also note that "it is important not to bureaucratize or co-opt what is essentially a grassroots movement."

REFERENCES

Alive and Kicking. (1991). [Television series]. United Kingdom: BBC Scotland.

Alcoholics Anonymous World Service. (1939). *Alcoholics Anonymous*. New York, NY: Works Publishing.

Best, D., Loaring, J., Ghufran, S., & Day, E. (2008, May 19). Different roads. *Drink and Drugs News*, p. 6. Retrieved from http://www.drinkanddrugsnews.com

Bryce, D. (2010). Voices of recovery. In R. Yates & M. Malloch (Eds.), *Tackling addiction: Pathways to recovery* (pp. 106–144). London, United Kingdom: Jessica Kingsley.

Bryce, D., & Pia, S. (2005). *Alive and kicking*. Edinburgh, Scotland: Mainstream.

Cloud, W., & Granfield, R. (2008). Conceptualizing recovery capital: Expansion of a theoretical construct. *Substance Use and Misuse, 43*, 1971–1986.

Faulkner, G., & Taylor, A. (Eds.). (2005). *Exercise, health, and mental health: Emerging relationships*. London, United Kingdom: Routledge.

Flint, J., Crawford, J., Parr, S., & Powell, R. (2010). *A process evaluation of Celtic Against Drugs and Rangers Positive Choices*. Edinburgh, Scotland: Scottish Government.

General Register Office for Scotland. (2010). *Life expectancy for administrative areas within Scotland, 2007–2009*. Edinburgh, Scotland: National Statistics Publication.

Gyarmathy, V., & Latkin, C. (2008). Individual and social factors associated with participation in treatment programs for drug users. *Substance Use and Misuse, 43*(12), 1865–1881.

Humphreys, K., King, S., McCarty, D., Chappel, J., Gallant, L., Haberle, B., . . . Weiss, R. (2004). Self-help organizations for alcohol and drug problems. *Journal of Substance Abuse Treatment, 26*, 151–158.

Kurtz, E. (1979). *Not-God: A history of Alcoholics Anonymous*. Center City, MN: Hazelden.

Laudet, A. (2007). What does recovery mean to you? Lessons from the recovery experience for research and practice. *Journal of Substance Abuse Treatment, 33*, 243–256.

MacDonald, A. (Producer), & Boyle, D. (Director) (1996). *Trainspotting* [Motion picture]. United Kingdom: Channel Four Films, Figment.

McKeganey, N., & McPike, M. (1997). *A process evaluation of Calton Athletics' drug prevention team*. Glasgow, Scotland: University of Glasgow.

Morgan, F. (1992, July 28). Calton Athletic faces closure. *Herald Scotland*. Retrieved from http://heraldscotland.com

Nutt, K. (2000, July 16). Fame turns sour in the drug war. *The Sunday Herald*. Retrieved from http://heraldscotland.com

Scotland's Futures Forum. (2008). *12 dimensions of a manageable problem: A collection of expert views*. Retrieved from http://www.scotlandfutureforum.org

Scottish Advisory Committee on Drug Misuse. (2008). *Essential care*. Edinburgh, Scotland: Author.

Scottish Government. (2008). *The road to recovery: A new approach to tackling Scotland's drug problem*. Edinburgh, Scotland: Author.

Scottish Government. (2009). *The road to recovery one year on*. Edinburgh, Scotland: Author.

UK Drug Policy Commission Recovery Consensus Group. (2008). *A vision of recovery*. London, United Kingdom: Author.

White, W., & Kurtz, E. (2005). *The varieties of recovery experience*. Chicago, IL: Great Lakes Addiction Technology Transfer Center.

White, W., & Kurtz, E. (2006). *Recovery: Linking addiction treatment and communities of recovery*. Northeast Pittsburgh, PA: Addiction Technology Transfer Center Network (ATTC).

Yates, R., & Malloch, M. (Eds.). (2010). *Tackling addiction: Pathways to recovery*. London, United Kingdom: Jessica Kingsley.

Serenity Café—on the Road to Recovery Capital

RUTH CAMPBELL

Comas, Edinburgh, Scotland, United Kingdom

KANE DUFFY, MICHAEL GAUGHAN, and MICHAEL MOCHRIE

Edinburgh, Scotland, United Kingdom

This story of the early-stage development of the Serenity Café with people recovering from addiction highlights the challenges and the possibilities for strengthening individual recovery through community development. Within the United Kingdom, the emphasis on treatment is beginning to make way for acknowledgement that social and community support following treatment is an important resource for sustaining recovery. However, we are somewhat short of practical and policy support for such ideas, although this, perversely, may allow for greater flexibility in the way the Serenity Café develops and may help engender empowerment to choose the terms of the process for those involved in recovery.

INTRODUCTION

This article has been developed by a group developing a recovery café in Edinburgh: a community development practitioner and three volunteers in recovery. It tells the story of a fledgling initiative in Edinburgh, Scotland. The Serenity Café is developing a hub for recovery-oriented social networks in Edinburgh. Although from inception it has aspired to become a 7-day café and recovery community focal point, it has developed to date as a virtual hub. It uses begged, borrowed, and rented space for diverse activities, a situation only mildly hindering the growth of the initiative which has been spurred on by volunteers in recovery.

The article starts with the Serenity Café story, illustrated with comments from volunteers and "customers" of the Serenity Café, gathered during a range of exercises. We then discuss the practice challenges and policy environment that are influencing our development. Finally, we reflect on what we have learned up to this point in our development. We hope practitioners and others can learn from our approach and will share theirs with us.

EVIDENCE

We use an action research approach in our work, while integrating investigative and evaluative exercises into our practice and inviting participants (people in recovery) to reflect with us on the findings. The exercises informing this article include:

- in-depth interviews during 2009 to 2010 in which we explored the recovery journeys (in this sample the majority attended a nonresidential, abstinence-focused treatment program) of nine volunteers, including seven males and two females, in recovery for varying periods of time from 8 months to 14 years and with addiction careers ranging from 15 to 30 years that include dependence on alcohol, opiates, psychostimulants, methadone maintenance prescription, and polysubstance use.
- two focus groups held in 2010 with 10 individuals (6 men and 4 women, ages 23 to 50+ years) who are customers of the Serenity Café.
- an online survey (97 responses) and three "customer feedback" surveys completed at Serenity Café events (171 responses), and comments from a review conducted with a first team of volunteers on their experience of being involved (14 responses), both during 2009.

We will add observations and anecdotes from our direct work with people involved. We feel these are legitimate as this is not a research article, but it is an illustrated discussion of our practice. In any work oriented toward helping people develop, what we learn on a day-to-day basis is an important source of evidence to determine what is working and what is not.

Throughout the article, we have drawn on a wide range of literature that has helped our thinking about the approach we are taking and helped us understand what is happening. Some of this literature is from the field of drug and alcohol practice and research, and some is from a wider range of disciplines including, importantly for us, community development, but it also draws on our experience of working with other disadvantaged groups in which resilience is a concept we find provides a useful framework for thinking about personal learning and development, a necessary component of the community development process.

We have also provided some contextual information on policy in Scotland relevant to recovery. In Scotland, we have a devolved government, and many hope that in the future this will allow us to forge a distinct path toward a more integrated, recovery-oriented, and community-led approach to meeting the needs of people contemplating and striving for recovery from addiction in Scotland. Hope, after all, is what we are all about.

THE SERENITY CAFÉ—THE BEGINNINGS

Motive

The Serenity Café began as a modest idea to establish a social enterprise by which a "high street" café would provide social space for people in recovery, while creating "first step" employment, traineeships, and volunteering opportunities for people in recovery trying to sustain abstinence. The social space would also provide a "nightclub" and be available to hold dances and functions. In many respects, there is nothing new here except the focus on recovery; many churches and voluntary organizations throughout the United Kingdom have trodden this path, with varying degrees of success. Comas, a small community development agency, set out to explore the possibilities of a recovery café.

The recovery focus followed the example of "sober nightclubs" and other facilities such as bookshops and cafés in the United States, which we saw promoted recovery openly and provided for people in recovery without the overly discreet, sometimes closeted image of mutual aid groups and their meeting places in our city. We wanted to promote positive opportunities for people to meet others in recovery and witness that happy, healthy recovery is possible and a viable, realistic life choice.

This open and celebratory approach reflected Comas's remit to promote social justice. City nightlife feels unsafe and unwelcoming to those of us who want a sober and drug-free social experience.

> New Year was a big problem for me. It was fantastic to go [to Serenity Café] because the entire town is drunk and it scares me. Having a place to go where I wasn't even thinking about alcohol made you relaxed about the whole thing. I was expecting to have a rubbish time. (Café customer)

Thinking about the practicalities of being in early recovery and trying to negotiate any form of "normal" social interaction in the evenings safely and without relapse triggers, we recognized that there was a real gap in availability of adult social venues that could be considered safe—safe in respect of being with others who shared the recovery experience and safe in respect of being "dry" and drug free. However, we also had a deep understanding of social exclusion. The lack of available dry and drug-free venues is part of a bigger problem. Drug users have been described as "multiply excluded and widely despised" (Ashton, 2008), and we found no reason to believe that giving up drugs or alcohol was a ticket to immediate social inclusion, for a number of reasons. Many alcohol and drug users have previously used substances to help them feel included and in recovery are having to form a new way of being in social environments. Although it is now increasingly documented that social support, and specifically social support for abstinence, is significant in the maintenance of recovery (Davis & Jason, 2005), there is a distinct lack of support available to people post-treatment, and particularly so outside the traditional public service hours of 9 am through 5 pm, Monday to Friday.

> Evenings are a big thing in early recovery, and weekends. Go to a meeting, get home at 9:30 pm, and I still look at the clock at [9:50 pm]. Because that's the time I would have to get to the off-license before it closes. And I still do it, still have that check. So I have to do something to distract myself. (Volunteer)

For many people, decades of social exclusion experienced during their addiction career have caused an erosion of social and coping skills, and for a significant number of people, addiction began in early life before a clear sense of self had fully formed. We saw a clear need to create opportunities in which people can form positive, supportive relationships, while "bridging" between the safe but somewhat cloistered environment of "the rooms" (mutual aid—Alcoholics Anonymous, Narcotics Anonymous, Cocaine Anonymous—fellowship meeting places) to wider social circles and social activities. We also saw a need to offer a positive alternative for those who do not find mutual aid fellowships meet their preferences.

> In early recovery then I would find it difficult to be around anyone drinking and even to be around my family members if I am honest. I think it is a great idea to have somewhere to go where you can just pop in and feel safe. (Community survey)

A further difference to a standard charitable enterprise, in addition to the recovery orientation, was the notion that the initiative should be developed and managed by people in recovery. From the outset, Comas sought to ensure that the "sense of ownership" was established as a necessary forerunner of actual ownership of the Serenity Café as a fully independent enterprise in the future, in keeping with the organization's community development ethos.

Initiation

To initiate the project, the first step toward developing the café idea was to check out with a broad spectrum of people in recovery whether the idea was of any interest at all. We developed an online survey and sent it through personal networks of people in recovery and asked them to snowball the link. Within a very short time, almost 100 people had responded—testament to the willingness and the networking capacity of people in recovery. We asked specific questions about people's potential use of a café for people in recovery; the questions were oriented toward assessing "market demand." Many respondents added "free text" comments expressing their need for a recovery-friendly venue. The response was overwhelmingly positive. Among the range of findings, 99% of respondents said they would use a recovery café and provided us with data on preferred opening hours, location, pricing, and preference for an openly recovery-oriented identity for the café; 70% of respondents said that meeting other people in recovery was important to their own recovery. People who provided their contact details in the survey and expressed a willingness to help were invited to an initial meeting. Only 2 people came! However, we persevered and established a steady attendance of around 10 people for four meetings.

Formation

It took time to establish relationships between people who came to the meetings and to form as a peer group. Recovery is a very loose common denominator in a group that can encompass very diverse people, leading to very different perspectives on the subject matter itself—what do we want from a café, and how will we set it up? Even though people had willingly come along to participate in discussions, the idea of the café was met with suspicion, doubt, and confusion, as well as great enthusiasm. Some people, particularly those in early recovery, found these meetings difficult and dropped out easily, but the grapevine surrounding mutual aid groups continued to serve us well and others came along. The format was informal group discussion with social breaks, with the aim of building an insight into the people who came along, their strengths, and what they might feel comfortable contributing to the development process.

At this stage, we began to fully appreciate the community development challenge we were facing. Business planning proved to be too abstract and challenging of a process for people to get their heads around. Within a very short space of time, we sensed that we needed to become action oriented as quickly as possible, or the suspicion and doubts would give way to defeatism. We were in danger of confirming for some people their fears that they did not know enough to make a contribution, the antithesis to our intentions.

We moved to a more experiential approach to provide more immediate rewards and opportunities to value different individual strengths by running some trial café-club nights to help reveal what other people in recovery in Edinburgh thought of the idea of a Serenity Café. Role modeling was provided by people in long-term recovery with some experience of community activism. With these people exerting the right balance of push and pull, the group attracted additional volunteers interested in a "hands-on" volunteering experience, and the first Serenity Café-Club night was launched, from a hired city center church hall. Nobody at this point knew what "success" looked like. Through fear of failure came solidarity between group members, but the buzz that came from running those first café club nights is still remembered by volunteers today. We would have been grateful if 50 people had come on that first night, but more than 100 came—and the same happened the next week and the next. The feedback from customers was endorsement of the idea and reward for the volunteers making it happen.

> I didn't think I would feel excited again, feel excited about doing something sober. (Café customer)

> I think it is just what the recovery community in Edinburgh has been lacking. Bring it on!! (Customer feedback)

> Fabulous idea. We need it! (Customer feedback)

Leadership and Teamwork

The need to manage and facilitate the group has always been demanding. "Teamwork" has not naturally emerged—there are "star roles" that are visible and attract attention from customers, from which some volunteers try to gain status and kudos, and there are lower-profile tasks, which tend to be neglected. The task is to continually ensure everyone is thanked and recognized equally, while providing room for reflection on personal progress as well as contribution to the team effort.

With no leadership naturally emerging from the group, the growing number of new volunteers attracted by the success of the events was not always effectively included in the process—with the self-absorbed nature of team members and the focus on the event itself, it became difficult to create a positive space for newcomers. The group readily proposed that leadership was needed, but no individual would take on this responsibility. In spite of regular training in leadership skills, this remains a difficult area. The group itself has come to recognize that "clean time" is not necessarily a predictor of leadership, but at the same time, we have learned the importance of guarding against "too much too soon" for people whose recovery is not so stable.

Volunteering and Recovery

Developing our approach to volunteering has been challenging. We found it is risky to single out individuals who appear to have potential and give them specific tasks key to the future of the project. Relying on one individual to "carry" a responsibility falls down when that individual decides a focus on recovery is more important to them at this point in their life (and we would always encourage that), or when, as we would hope, their growing confidence leads them to go to college or start a new job. For others, stepping back from involvement with the Serenity Café has also been a protection against relapse (avoiding too much stress); others have stepped back from involvement because of mental illness (a number of our volunteers have been ascribed a "dual diagnosis"). So we have retained a focus on working collectively as much as possible. We devised a peer mentoring program in which people more experienced in volunteering with the Serenity Café are matched with new volunteers. A move toward structured volunteering plans for individuals, in which they set goals for what they want to achieve from volunteering, has helped initiate an explosion of new activity led by volunteers, in ways that had not occurred when volunteering was a more casual arrangement. The explicit personal goals, together with logging volunteer hours and a process of peer mentor support and feedback, helped transform the volunteering toward a much more focused use of volunteer time.

Sustaining Momentum

The continuation of the café-club nights on a monthly basis has had both positive and negative effects on development. Positively, we rapidly became part of a "recovery scene" in Edinburgh, and this brought positive relationships that have grown toward informal partnership with some service providers, discussed later. This in turn has brought us to the attention of policymakers and potential suppliers of funding, which may lead to realization of our ambitions. Ambitions, indeed, have grown a great deal since the original conception of a recovery-oriented café. The Serenity Café is now conceived as a "recovery hub" for Edinburgh and houses any aspect of social, cultural, and learning opportunities and support, which users want to generate. Valentine similarly describes his experience in the United States: "a recovery-oriented anchor in the hearts of the communities, a place where local communities of recovery can design and deliver the supports they need to initiate and maintain their recovery" (White, 2007, p. 83). A Serenity Café football team has emerged, a women's group has begun, and volunteer-led activity groups range from a drama club to fishing and golf.

On the downside, energy and focus have easily been drawn toward the café-club nights to the extent that interest in planning for the longer term diminished to dangerously low levels. In part, this may have been due to lack of confidence, in which volunteers opt for hands-on, practical tasks rather than the more cerebral approach required for planning and strategizing. In part, it may be due to the lack of modeling available to people in recovery who have not had previous involvement in community activism.

Nurturing Grassroots Action

We considered carefully how to rebuild interest in steering the overall long-term development. It appeared to us essential that we valued potential and not experience. Although tempting at times, we did not want to install a higher echelon of people in recovery who are professionals with the skills and experience to easily form a token committee, to lead the process. We felt a more genuine empowerment could come from demonstrating that people whose addiction careers started at an early age—cutting them off from learning and employment—and who are now in recovery can learn, develop, and achieve their full potential with the right opportunities. Our challenge has been to ensure that volunteers see the task of developing the Serenity Café as the right kind of opportunity.

> I need community involvement and a sense of purpose. The Serenity Café feels like inclusion and a feeling of giving something back. (Volunteer)

It takes care and practice to facilitate a process by which everyone's contribution is valued, and tasks and support are tailored to provide progressive stepping stones of just the right height for different individuals which leads toward increased self-esteem and self-efficacy and can then lead to positive engagement with positions of responsibility within the Serenity Café steering group—no matter what a person brings in the way of formal qualifications or experience.

> In the planning committee our ideas are listened to, you feel you are making a contribution and you feel valued. (Volunteer)

We hope that as the community development process behind the Serenity Café becomes clearer, it will create interest in recovery community development, which in turn might strengthen our capacity in Scotland to promote more collective action and strengthen the recovery community. We are in the process of designing vocational qualifications in recovery community development to accredit volunteers' work. Ward (2000, p. 49) described empowerment practice as work that "encourages and enables people to try out and experience new ways of influencing their life chances," and which we believe in the Serenity Café works in parallel with the mutually beneficial process of helping others in recovery. As Bamber (2009b, p. 4) points out, community "is the one thing that systems cannot produce," so we feel that an important part of the learning from the Serenity Café relates to the challenges of working to develop the capacity of a group of people in recovery to work collectively for a community goal.

Community Leadership and Community Development—the Steering Group

> Serenity Café gave me responsibility. Addicts don't cope with that very well; I would have run a mile from that in the past. (Volunteer)

We have avoided for as long as possible the formalization of a "committee" and the imposition of any particular approach to decision making. Decision-making structures work best when they fit with existing cultural systems, of which mutual aid fellowships are the most familiar to the majority of our volunteers. We tend to agree with Burns and Taylor (1998) that people in excluded communities tend not to be natural "joiners" of community groups because of their history and sense of alienation and are often suspicious of formalization and emergence of leaders. In the 1st year of the Serenity Café, we saw a very dynamic process in which around 40 people were involved in volunteering in various ways, but a small core of 5 have sustained their involvement from the outset. Within this period, some people have given short-term but significant contributions that have moved the group forward while using the opportunity for their own development. Some volunteers were self-protective and naturally reluctant to invest a lot of commitment and energy in something that initially, it seemed, had a reasonably high risk for failure. Certainly, once the Serenity Café had shown it could be successful, more people began to get involved. In addition to reluctance to put themselves forward, once engaged, trying to form a steering group of people in recovery was very challenging and has required a major investment of time in supporting individuals to take on roles and make a contribution.

It has been challenging to find an approach that suits volunteers with diverse interests, experiences, and temperaments. Those who do need structure become easily frustrated by those who need flexibility, yet each can learn from the other if the timing is right. We discuss later the personal development process within volunteers' engagement with the development of the Serenity Café and the different starting points that different individuals have come along with. We have not set a threshold for length of time in recovery before a volunteer can join the steering group. We have learned during the last year that not everyone is ready for the responsibility of being on a steering group, and those who appear ready are not necessarily on a uniform and linear process of personal development. Their personal peaks and troughs can lead to erratic attendance, and with this, the steering group is only very slowly developing maturity. Paterson, Weaver, and Crawford (2010) noted that some addictions therapists regard "user involvement" as potentially counter-therapeutic and as exposing "vulnerable users to stressful situations" (p. 92). Although we do not regard our approach as "user involvement" per se, our experience confirms that in some cases participation can be stressful for individuals. However, empowerment cannot take place if there is a fundamental belief that addiction and recovery are hopeless states, nor can it take place in environments where people are infantilized. We would suggest that empowering people in recovery is a fundamental aspect of raising our national game in supporting people in addiction and recovering from addiction and has become the *raison d'etre* of the Serenity Café. To empower people is not to avoid risk or challenge, but it must involve ensuring an appropriate climate for people to engage in discussion and sufficient individual support for people to gain learning and development from the collective process.

> The guidance and support during volunteering was an important part for me—I'm in early recovery and at times feel anxious. The support was caring and genuine and I was made to feel part of the team. (Volunteer review)

Empowerment cannot properly take place unless a group becomes consciously engaged in discussion and decision making—as practitioners, we must constantly be wary of making decisions ourselves with the best of intentions to maintain momentum or respond to outside pressures though thinking groups are "not ready for it." The pressure to present a viable proposition to funders and evidence success to policymakers could easily tempt us to cut corners. Group maturity allows for constructive argument about those aspects of running the Serenity Café that will require thorough debate and must be made by the group itself, such as employing staff and formalizing volunteering, ethical positions on sponsorship, and funding. We have also found there is a need to stress the importance of bringing discussion to the full group. The success of the Serenity Café has encouraged some individuals to derive personal status from acting "on behalf" of the group without the collective delegation of authority to do so. Clear boundaries are important. Debate and complex solution finding to the challenges we will no doubt face in the realization of our ambitions will require volunteers to think beyond themselves and their own needs, which in turn may require a level of personal maturity to disagree without dismissing others' views.

THE PRACTICE CHALLENGES

Personal Development and Community Development

> I don't want to just recover from dependencies; I want to recover from behaviors. I want the old me to be dead, safely in the past. (Volunteer)

Reflecting on our work during the last year, we suggest that personal development and community development are inextricably linked in what we do. Individual learning and development is coupled with and mutually reinforced by the process of peer support and the reciprocity within helping relationships. The strengthening of individual social networks of support in turn creates and reinforces a sense of community, and the building of personal recovery capital contributes to and strengthens the collective recovery capital available to the community. This in turn can be used to make stronger demands on national resources for recovery.

> One big word for Serenity Café is 'opportunity.' I don't want to sound like 'Captain Cliché,' but it is opportunity for growth in lots of ways. (Volunteer)

It is the responsibility of all community practitioners to purposefully create the right conditions for personal learning and development. However, we have developed far more of a focus in this project on the individual processes involved than would be typical in a community development process. We have mentioned that individual characteristics of the people in recovery we are working with make the work challenging. Within the Serenity Café, our lack of staff capacity to really build and strengthen this area of our work has been one of our greatest frustrations, and we take the work extremely seriously. We do not want the cost of success to be counted in relapses or individuals further experiencing a sense of exclusion within this group. We are slowly building a peer support process that typically happens naturally between some volunteers but that does not happen naturally for some who have personal characteristics or complex needs requiring a more deliberate and planned process of peer support. We are very aware of the vulnerability of people particularly in early recovery when they are raw and balancing wild enthusiasm for their new recovery with muddled thinking, emotional swings, and for many, a brittleness and immaturity as if adolescence has come back to haunt bodies that give the outward impression of being adult.

> There is a need for accessible support by the service users/volunteers within the setting and knowledge of addictions/recovery by staff. (Community survey)

> Once I was clean and sober, a huge amount of issues emerged that had been hidden by addiction. (Volunteer)

> I have paralyzing days where I'm off my trolley. I've pushed it all down for so long, things like a friend's death 10 years ago I had never come to terms with; alcohol took it all away. (Volunteer)

The Serenity Café's growing relationship with a local treatment center means the café-club events are visited by people while in treatment, in turn encouraging some to come forward as volunteers upon leaving treatment. We are therefore close witnesses to people's first adaptations to life in recovery. Many people have grown up with a way of being that is hard to leave behind. Kemp (2009) describes the means by which people become profoundly lonely during addiction, in ways in which simply "being around" other people does not penetrate. He points out that society's attitude to addicts has throughout the years of people's addiction careers been embodied within the individual as a deep sense of personal shame, out of which comes sensitivity to rejection, dishonor, or aggression. What we see in the Serenity Café is a very fragile growth of social relationships forged through the common bond of running the café-club events and other Serenity Café activities and working toward achieving our long-term ambitions.

> You have to work for personal growth. I was emotionally raw. I was nuts! The scariest part of my life was the first few months of recovery. (Volunteer)

> I didn't even know what I liked doing, no idea who or what I was … might sound really dull and silly to some people, but before this, I had never read a whole book, and I love it! (Volunteer)

Resilience and Attachment in Personal Development

While we are very privileged to see people blossom and experience pride and joy in their recovery, we must also take responsibility for giving this the best possible chance of budding and then being sustained into mature growth. This has led us to draw on Comas's experience of working to build resilience in individuals. The comments from volunteers and what we have learned during the last year suggest the concept of resilience is highly relevant to people in recovery. Resilience encompasses three main principles of attachment, self-esteem, and self-efficacy—or more plainly, "I have," "I am," and "I can."

"Attachment" is a common theme in child and family social work and early education, in which a child's secure attachment predicts stronger coping mechanisms and freedom to learn, based on a strong bond between the child and significant adult. What we often see among Serenity Café volunteers is the adult outcome of insecure attachment, because many people have experienced poor family backgrounds or childhood trauma, which as we all know is a commonly documented factor among people with addictions. What this means in practice is that the building of social networks between people and the development of peer support is a tricky business. A number of volunteers exemplify different attachment styles—avoidant, ambivalent, and chaotic attachment styles—which require us to respond to individuals differently but also challenge us to facilitate and support group dynamics to ensure the Serenity Café hangs together as a collective process. Individual attachment is not a marginal concern within community development. Communities are formed through social relationships, which in turn nurture shared purpose and encourage commitment to the hard work of achieving goals together. Although it is challenging to provide the support demanded from some of the more insecure individuals, the understanding by more experienced volunteers in recovery, of the confusing nature of early recovery, can bring a patience and tolerance that are hard to find elsewhere. We provide an opportunity for people to freely give of themselves and contribute to the well-being of the community as a whole, a process through which volunteers gain an appreciation of their own self-worth and complete a virtuous circle. However, we have observed that many of the volunteers who appear to be making good progress in their recovery have a secure attachment figure, a relative, partner, or friend, who has been with them through "thick and thin" and is still offering love and acceptance. Volunteers who struggle with recovery tend to be people who are more isolated but for whom building supportive relationships is a difficult task—people who, if in mutual aid groups, regularly "sack" their sponsors, flit from one personal development fad to another without settling into a belonging, and within the Serenity Café, blow hot and cold with their commitment and relating to others.

> I've never had a healthy relationship with women, and it's terrifying doing things sober for the first time. (Volunteer)

> I feel really behind a lot of people the same age as me, kind of emotionally stunted. (Volunteer)

Being involved in a social environment such as the Serenity Café, which promotes a climate of honesty and self-awareness, is one way for people to start to form relationships.

Self-Care and Self-Knowledge

A further concept we are integrating into our work with volunteers is what Neff (2009, p. 212), an educational psychologist, calls "self-compassion," which she proposes offers the benefits of high self-esteem "without the downsides." She describes self-compassion as "(a) self-kindness versus self-judgment, (b) a sense of common humanity versus isolation, and (c) mindfulness versus over-identification." What we like about this is that we recognize that the experience of many of our volunteers is indeed a hyperattention to their flaws and mistakes. Those in longer-term recovery often seem to have a greater ability to accept their real humanity, failings, flaws, and all and get on with loving life anyway.

> I was so sick and tired of being the person I was. I don't want to hate myself, I want to forgive myself. That is what I want for me, which is why I do so much. (Volunteer)

> In the [throes] of addiction, your perception of self isn't reality; it's distorted. (Volunteer)

> Forced to accept the reality of who you were. Admit mistakes and apologize. Far less bullshit. Far less 'I am.' I still exaggerate, there's still a part of me that thinks I'm special. Now I think I'm worth it rather than think I'm special. (Volunteer)

Neff (2009, p. 213) suggests that self-compassion is strongly associated with psychological well-being and "increased feelings of happiness, optimism, curiosity and connectedness, as well as decreased anxiety, depression, rumination and fear of failure ... [self-compassion is] associated with greater personal initiative to make needed changes in one's life." This appears to be a good fit with the process of supporting personal development in recovery, particularly for people without secure relationships in their life who may feel bereft of others' compassion. As yet, we are simply using an awareness of self-compassion in our dialogue with people, the way we approach group discussion when things have not gone as well as expected, and in presenting ourselves as role models—flawed human beings but nevertheless cheerfully keeping on.

> Gaining hope opened the door, hearing what other people had been through and seeing them integrate into society and able to laugh. (Volunteer)

Self-efficacy is also a concept used in helping professions, but in environments promoting recovery, it requires careful thought. As Bandura (2006) points out, efficacy in different realms of functioning is not necessarily transferable. When working with people in early recovery, we are in fact working with people who feel quite de-skilled, whose strategies, skills, and tactics for getting on in the drug-using or drinking community are not automatically helping them to negotiate a niche for themselves in the wider social world that has been rejecting them for so long. What we are doing in the Serenity Café is providing a range of different opportunities to use skills positively and to develop and practice new skills until people feel confident they can take these skills into new environments.

Not much over a year ago, handling all that cash behind the bar, that would have been in my pocket. Serenity Café gave me responsibility; addicts don't cope with that very well. I would have run a mile from that in the past. (Volunteer)

Mutual Gain

One aspect of the Serenity Café widely recognized as beneficial is that of allowing people to "give something back" in a helping role. Gartner and Reissman's (1979) conceptualization of helping as a process that reinforces a person's own learning and strengthens their positive attitudes, values, and skills is something we feel strongly aligned to within the Serenity Café. However, this is a long-term process for some individuals—tasks can be done selfishly or in the spirit of sharing, and it is our task to help people overcome their tendency toward self-absorption and to begin to feel part of a team rather than an individual with a single focus on their own task. The development of a stronger sense of teamwork requires some deliberate work at enabling people to appreciate others' contributions at every opportunity. We do not have a ritualistic reflection at the end of each event, but we do want to design some kind of process by which volunteers can be supported to express appreciation of what others contribute.

It's such an incremental process, you're not always aware of your own progress. You're able to do things you might never have been able to do. (Volunteer)

Finally, what we most obviously help individuals to develop, both for volunteers and customers of the Serenity Café, is social networks. Best, Ghufran, Day, Rajashree, and Loaring (2008) identified that "factors associated with maintaining [...] abstinence were linked more often to social networks, including moving away from heroin-using friends and relying on support from non-using friends" (p. 623). At the beginning of the Serenity Café, the single most obvious driver was that a safe, drink- and drug-free adult social environment is needed. It was corroborated first in our community survey, then by customer feedback.

All the places I used to go are off limits now; I need somewhere to relax with other people in recovery. (Community survey)

In early recovery, I didn't have the confidence to phone people up. Meetings and the Serenity Café are a bridge to build up social skills. (Café customer)

> Phoning is not as easy as walking into a café. You don't want to talk about what's wrong; you just want to be with someone. (Café customer)

Some people identify that social contact is an important factor in overcoming their emotional fragility and potential for self-isolation, while others recognize that recovery comes with loss of previous social circles associated with drinking and drug use. For some people, others in recovery become a support network that replaces lost family relationships.

Modeling Happy, Healthy, and Fulfilled Recovery

Another hugely important factor for people in early recovery, and people who come as customers of the Serenity Café while still in treatment, is the positive image of a social life in recovery.

> Dancing at the Serenity Café while sober was the best day of my life; I woke up the next day full of this thought that I had done that. (Volunteer)

Many people have entered recovery assuming that abstinence is the end of a social life, and in Scottish culture, this perception would be reinforced in any mainstream social circle, from teenage years on.

> You meet so many people tripping over their bottom lip, but recovery can be fun. I thought my life was over when I had to put down substances. I thought I can't do this or that, can't go to a nightclub. An aspect of that is true because of the nature of my recovery. But Serenity Café gives you something. My nieces and nephews thought I was really sad as though I had to sit in at nights behind a locked door. When they heard about Serenity Café and that you get a wee boogie, they thought it was great. It's like in the story, do you have to go around wearing the chains of past sins? It doesn't have to be like that—it's to be enjoyed, not endured. (Volunteer)

> It's got me living again, not just feeling sorry for myself because I can't be like a normal person and drink. (Café customer)

As we have seen, working in ways that meet the needs of individuals in recovery is a basic building block of working with them to feel a sense of belonging to a community and to participate effectively in a development process. As in individual helping relationships, the opportunity to be involved in a development process brings additional benefits to individuals that individualized therapeutic approaches might sometimes lack, while the collecting of aspirations brings benefit to the wider identity and purpose of a recovery community. However, the concept of a "recovery community" is not yet clearly defined in Scotland.

Mutual Aid—Live and Let Thrive

> I see people get through incredible things in meetings, and they don't pick up. (Volunteer)

The Serenity Café experience reflects the positive principles established over many years by mutual aid groups. Folgheraiter and Pasani (2009, p. 265) found evidence that self-help and mutual aid groups do help to "regenerate social relationships and therefore the well-being and quality of life of local communities," forming a social capital that bridges people from a negative past to positive citizenship.

The Serenity Café would not have been possible without the existence of a growing and thriving mutual aid scene in Edinburgh. The clear and positive message within mutual aid of "giving service" and peer support has contributed to the Serenity Café ethos. And yet not everyone in mutual aid has welcomed or "approved of" the Serenity Café either. The Serenity Café has still to fully come to terms with its relationship with Edinburgh's mutual aid community. One feature that has caused the most excitement and the most disdain is our focus on recovery, not on the substance. Many are thrilled that Serenity Café has succeeded in bringing "people from different fellowships together," while others have maintained their separatist preferences.

> I would be deeply offended by any hint of affiliation with Narcotics Anonymous. (Community survey)

> Strong affiliations with one fellowship could prove to be off-putting. I feel that something like this is long overdue in a capital city and this is a fantastic time to start it. There appears to be a strong recovery community emerging with healthy crossover between fellowships; therefore, it would be fantastic to have a neutral meeting place. (Community survey)

As many will know, the traditions of 12-step mutual aid groups forbid affiliation or endorsement of any outside bodies. There is no doubt that the word-of-mouth networking facilitated during the minutes before and after mutual aid meetings has served the Serenity Café very well in terms of reaching the wider recovery community, but we have been careful to ensure volunteers avoid direct marketing of café-club events at meetings. Some "traditionalists" have objected to enthusiasts sharing their experience of the Serenity Café as part of their personal testimony during meetings, which is not something we have encouraged, but we also cannot discourage it—their personal testimony is their own. Some have suggested that the Serenity Café is planning to make a profit out of recovery, to which we have responded with very clear and transparent explanations of how the Serenity Café might attract funds, generate income from the café, and dedicate all funds to further developing opportunities for people in recovery. The Serenity Café does not favor any particular treatment method or path to sustained recovery. We have volunteers who have never been in treatment and managed their recovery entirely through mutual aid, and we have volunteers who have been in treatment and never attended or felt attracted by 12-step mutual aid groups. However, the fact is that the majority of our volunteers and café customers do also attend mutual aid groups. Some mutual aid traditions have spilled over into the Serenity Café, such as a great deal of hugging, which to the nonhuggers among us has taken some getting used to. We celebrate "birthdays" (anniversaries of becoming sober/drug free). We have developed in a way that is sensitive to people's "need" for meetings and have accepted the precedence a "home group" will take over a Serenity Café planning meeting.

However, we do feel the need to be deliberate about creating a positive and welcoming atmosphere that respects *everyone's* recovery journey, no matter how it has been taken and no matter what stage of the journey someone is on. The task is to represent recovery positively and in a celebratory way.

> A fantastic idea and a great way to eradicate recovery fascism. (Customer feedback)

We have developed enormous respect for the accessibility and durability of the mutual aid movement, but sadly, we also encounter a great deal of prejudice toward it among other professionals involved in drug and alcohol treatment, among funders, and in policy circles. Much of this based on a great deal of ignorance about the way mutual aid groups work, which seems to be an unfortunate side effect of those groups' traditions on nonaffiliation. This challenges us to think carefully and act ethically—to help counter the negative attitudes we encounter while ensuring that our own open position is understood and respected. Unfortunately, part of the problem we face is that the massive contribution of mutual aid groups to recovery in Scotland is not yet recognized within policies concerning recovery in Scotland.

> There's no possibility I'm using tomorrow. I've learned what I have to do [through mutual aid group]; I've been through pain, anger; I've learned I can get through what life throws at me as long as I do what I need to do. (Volunteer)

THE POLICY CONTEXT

Empowerment is a political as well as an individual and community process. We have trained steering group members on how policymaking and the political process works. They have challenged government ministers in person, written a recovery manifesto for all the political parties to consider in their development of party manifestos in advance of the next general election, and are becoming more astute and active members of policy fora at the local and national levels. This has required significant individual support. Serenity Café representatives have been directly challenged by professionals who are wary of promoting abstinent recovery. It is hard for people in recovery to be among large groups of professionals and even more difficult not to take such challenges very personally.

Several areas of Scottish policy particularly concern the development of the Serenity Café—policies relating to alcohol and drug addiction, policies relating to mental health, and policies relating to employability and trends in third sector funding. Serenity Café volunteers cannot be everywhere at once to meet the demands of policymakers for "user involvement" in all of these spheres in which, in any case, they would be responding to others' agendas rather than setting their own. A balance has to be struck between gaining a profile at the national policymaking level and getting on with the grassroots action.

Drugs

The debate in Scotland about addiction focuses largely on drugs. Media attention is a strong driver focusing attention on the cost of addiction and the cost of treatment. The public, at least, expects that a "value for money" outcome of public service intervention might be that a person becomes drug or alcohol free and stays that way. In the wake of a national news channel's pointed assertion that the "success rate" of drug treatment (reported in an English study) may only be 3%, a battle began in the "drugs and addictions" press about the purpose of treatment, and commentators weighed in with polarized views, as one might expect.

There is no doubt that Scottish policy is slowly turning toward recovery, but slow is the operative word. Scotland's policy statement on drugs is called the *Road to Recovery* (Scottish Government, 2009b) but the policy is still dominated by treatment—McKeganey (2008) is right (on this point at least): The target setting following the *Road to Recovery* in 2008 did focus on getting more people into treatment, not on the actual outcome of treatment. Within the Serenity Café, we have argued that after investing in treatment, it makes sense to secure that investment by supporting a range of opportunities to strengthen recovery and prevent relapse. Compared with the cost of treatment, an initiative like the Serenity Café looks almost too cheap to be real, as it is based on a strong ethic of self-help and volunteering. Yet it will be hard for us to make justifiable demands for public sector support for the Serenity Café unless we can evidence the obvious case that relapse costs, and investment in supporting long-term recovery represents a positive saving. The government has chosen not to impose the measurement of long-term outcomes after treatment on services for the time being.

Alcohol

A further difficulty for the Serenity Café is that the development of drugs policy in Scotland has remained determinedly separate from alcohol policy. We are recovery oriented not substance oriented. While the problem of addiction has always been central to drugs policy, it has been harder for alcohol policies to "place" recovery, which involves abstinence as a desirable goal, because the alcohol policy itself (Scottish Government, 2008a) has been almost too polite (or too much in thrall to the alcohol lobby) to dwell on alcoholism. To some extent, the experience of people in the Serenity Café reflects this, where people addicted to alcohol appear to have had far more short-term hospital admissions and detoxes with no support for recovery offered on discharge (and after which most freely admit they drank within hours) and a far more circuitous route into treatment compared with those whose main addiction was to drugs. Qualitative data from our individual interviews with volunteers suggest that there has been much more of a lottery for alcoholics in relation to the chances of meeting staff within general practice, community mental health services, or psychiatric services who have any understanding or skills to work with their addiction. Drug treatment appears to offer a much more visible and accessible range of services and staff with specialized training and experience, supporting self-referral by users as well as agency-assisted referral.

The separation of drugs and alcohol policy is also marked by the recent establishment by the Scottish Government of a national Recovery Consortium for drugs, an important milestone for recovery in Scotland but missing an important chance to focus on recovery, not on the substance.

Mental Health Recovery

In relation to policies concerning mental health, we will not go into too much detail here. We have learned from the recovery movement in mental health, which permeates national policy and community-based practice in this field. We have recently become aware of a tendency by public health managers to conflate strategies for promoting mental health recovery, which has been well funded and supported for several years, and addictions recovery in the manner of "here's one we made earlier." This is no doubt driven by a lack of resources but overlooks a fundamental principle of community development and user involvement, in which people directly affected by addiction (and indeed addiction and mental health issues) should be the ones who decide whether they fall in with mental health recovery, or whether they explore issues for themselves and lead development in the direction they decide is appropriate for them. To present only one path is not a choice. We are not proponents of reinventing wheels, but we should take the time to design a round wheel rather than use a square one designed for another purpose—although we may learn much about wheel design from the square one.

Employability and Welfare

In the current climate of welfare reform, employability will become an even more critical area affecting many people recovering from addiction. Policies on drugs, alcohol, and employability all recognize that employment can help people to sustain their recovery, and there is research to support this proposition. It is true that when we initially explored the idea of the Serenity Café, the potential for employing people in recovery, or creating traineeships for them, was high on our list of "selling points" for the idea. We have not lost this vision, but we have tempered it with a much more realistic sense of what is really involved in the journey toward employability for people in early recovery in the Serenity Café.

The task of finding employment for people after leaving treatment is often viewed simplistically. McKeganey and McIntosh's (2006) critique of a project trying to support people from addiction to employability described it as a confusion between "... an employment project for ex and recovering drug users that has an element of therapy and support added in, or a therapeutic project for drug users that contains an element of employment support." This appears to overlook the very real challenges we have observed people in early recovery experiencing when, as we have already discussed, people are unsure of who they are, never mind in which direction they are going. Bamber (2009a, p. 4) describes the challenge well: "The suggestion that the construction and reconstruction of identity is something that can be delivered by services is a profound misunderstanding of this process ... [what is needed is to] embed individuals who choose to change in environments conducive to identity reconstruction and personal growth." What we feel the Serenity Café offers is an opportunity for people to try different experiences that help them construct their new identity as a person in recovery, with associated feelings of self-efficacy with which to take on new challenges in terms of further education or employment. This is not a simple question of either creating employment in a recovery-oriented environment or of a process creating employment-ready individuals to meet whatever skills gap the government has recently identified. Beyond a recovery-oriented environment, potential employees are disadvantaged by prejudice against their past, which may include a criminal record and long gaps in employment history, if there is any history at all. Even if employers were enlightened, as Banjoko points out (as cited in Craig, 2008): "It's the characteristics of ex-users that make it hard for them to find and keep work—the stresses and strains of work often lead them to revert to familiar coping mechanisms. Much will depend on the ex-user prior to their drug usage . . . above all, support networks are needed, and long-term support in particular" (p. 13). We are aware of the preferences of public sector commissioners to seek programs that process people through short-term programs into a state of job readiness, which has led to a range of projects in the employability field pressured by targets that they meet by screening potential project candidates rigorously to reduce the possibility of failure. This is not a climate in which vulnerable people receive individually appropriate, long-term support.

There are further complications in the United Kingdom (welfare benefits policy is not devolved to Scotland's government), where there is a move to push benefit claimants from "welfare to work," which brings new pressures on people in the Serenity Café. Welfare benefits provide a safety net and a very real safe haven for people in recovery in the form of housing benefit. In Edinburgh, there is enlightened effort by housing officials to support people to leave treatment and move into new neighborhoods, enabling people to cut ties with their substance-using past. The pressure on social housing locally has prompted a pragmatic approach to using private landlords to house social housing applicants and using welfare benefits to pick up the tab. In practice, this reinforces the disincentive to find work, because the private rents would be too steep to be covered by minimum wage, should the tenant find work. Some volunteers use Disability Living Allowance (a state benefit awarded to people with chronic illness or disability to help with care and mobility and is independent of employment or unemployment) to support their transition to further learning at college or work, although it is ironic that people are forced to revert to highlighting their incapacity to build their capacity and strengthen their recovery.

So, the Serenity Café must take care about the claims it makes and the goals it sets for itself in relation to employability and must ensure that we insist on a holistic approach and provide practical support for people in all aspects of their lives so that all the building blocks toward a future in employment stack up. With the national push to get people into treatment, we can assume that the age of people in recovery will be getting younger—indeed the youngest involved in the Serenity Café are in their early 20s—so it is important that we do encourage career aspirations. At the same time, we must ensure that any employment we do offer creates a viable opportunity for those who feel they are caught in a benefits trap, as well as a genuinely supportive environment in which to develop.

Third Sector Funding—Social Enterprise Myth and Reality

The Serenity Café is developing in the midst of a recession, placing severe pressure on every aspect of life, from consumer spending to public services and including the charitable sector. It is not the best time to be considering starting a new enterprise. Established drugs and alcohol agencies are experiencing grant cuts, and we may face a backlash if we are given a leg up by public sector funders at this time. Funds from all potential sources are increasingly scarce as philanthropic bodies' giving reflects low interest rates on their endowments.

One answer increasingly being promoted in the United Kingdom as a means of creating opportunity is social enterprise. This has become the mantra in central government approaches to the third sector, with all new investment channeled toward making the charitable and community sector more business-like and self-sustaining. The Scottish Social Enterprise Coalition declares that social enterprise is "the deal which delivers independence, unrestricted income and long term sustainability" (Swanson, 2009, p. 9)—rhetoric the government seems to have fallen for hook, line, and sinker.

Again, at the beginning of our journey, we assumed that we could play this game, with a well-planned business model that would show that the Serenity Café could generate sufficient income from café sales to operate as a viable enterprise. We were wrong. We realized very quickly that most high-street cafés survive because they operate on a skeleton staff and waste no money on supporting people or providing supervised developmental opportunities for volunteers.

> Possibly need a supervisor-type person to go round at regular intervals making sure everyone was OK. (Volunteer review)

> "Would like more support re: time out on the night. (Volunteer review)

When we approached an organization specifically established with government help to support social enterprises, we found the emphasis to be entirely on enterprise—the "social" in social enterprise apparently only window dressing for an approach that has mistakenly reduced the complex challenges in the third sector financing of services and support for vulnerable people to a simple lack of business sense. We were advised that we should push up prices to boost sales figures—a move we cannot contemplate if we are to attract vulnerable people in early recovery who are on welfare benefits—and reduce the number of staff we anticipate are needed to provide for the personal development and recovery support of workers, volunteers, and customers in recovery. We are not willing to undervalue the potential of the Serenity Café to transform lives and promote recovery.

> A lot of these guys are still on benefits, and it can be very expensive to meet up in most cafés and have a snack or a coffee; it would be a great benefit if they had somewhere to socialize that was more affordable to their budget. Learning to socialize and being able to do so in a relaxed and safe environment is important to people's recovery. (Community survey)

The Serenity Café faces a number of challenges in becoming a viable concern that is as self-sustaining as possible. The extortionate cost of premises in Edinburgh prices out of the market enterprises with a focus on social need. Our work with volunteers during the last year has demonstrated that creating a supportive and positive environment in which employees, trainees, and volunteers can strengthen their recovery and flourish as individuals, while creating a recovery hub for the growing recovery community, requires significant staff time, which may not be possible to recoup through café sales to a target market largely reliant on state benefits for their spending power. We have been encouraged by the comments of customers ("There should be one in every city," customer feedback) and requests for advice from many other parts of the United Kingdom seeking to learn from and develop a local Serenity Café. Creating a replicable model is important to us. While we can gather evidence of the social impact of what we are doing, it will take longer for us to say confidently that there is a working financial model behind it. But replication need not be about creating carbon-copy initiatives—it is about taking the best of what we do and applying principles where these are relevant.

At present, we think a hybrid funding model—social enterprise with grant aid—is the required formula, which is not quite business-like enough for some and not looking quite enough like a recognizable service (i.e., treatment service) for others. We anticipate that even with funding support in the coming years, full user-led operation as an independent entity may take several years to achieve. Our task is to ensure that potential funders recognize and support that development timescale.

Finding a Policy Niche for the Serenity Café—Abstinent Recovery

At present then, Serenity Café is somewhat outside the sphere of policymakers and falls between several policy domains, in particular, between the separation in drugs and alcohol policies.

One important aspect of both drugs and alcohol policy and the prevailing culture among practitioners in Scotland is difficulty with the term "abstinence." *The Road to Recovery* (Scottish Government, 2008b) describes recovery as "a process through which an individual is enabled to move on from their problem drug use, towards a drug free life as an active and contributing member of society" (p. vi). After stating the need to move beyond an artificial distinction between harm reduction and abstinence, the chapter on recovery steadfastly avoids using the "A" word again.

We have found that using the word abstinence provokes quite hostile reactions from practitioners in the drug field, no doubt a throwback from 30 years ago when many of us fought valiantly for harm reduction to be recognized as a legitimate and pragmatic approach to the challenges we faced with the emergence of blood-borne viruses including HIV. We continue to acknowledge the importance of harm reduction as an approach and acknowledge that many people involved in the Serenity Café owe their recovery to a period of maintenance prescribing, which allowed them to stabilize their lives and consider their long-term goals. Interestingly, many of our volunteers and participants report that their drug workers did not discuss goals and certainly did not encourage them to think that abstinence was achievable, in some cases actively discouraging reducing dosage. This experience is also borne out in other research studies, as Best, Groshkova, and McTague (2009) reports: "For clients who aspire to change, the system is often poorly articulated and structured to succeed … organisational cultures [. . .] often do not believe in recovery and which tend to be sceptical of clients' claims for abstinence." Valentine described a period in the development of a community of recovery in the United States in which this attitude was first perceived as a threat by those working in treatment. It eventually calmed down when it was recognized there was no actual competition (as quoted in White, 2007).

It appears in Scotland we will have to continue to explain that there is a place for abstinence in the vocabulary of recovery. We have been directly and indirectly steered away from using the term by potential funders, and yet not using the word to describe the recovery of the people using the Serenity Café would seem to be selling them short, because their abstinence is what they take pride in and what they perceive as keeping them alive.

CREATING COLLABORATIVE ADVANTAGE

Partnership Working

> I wonder what it would be like to harness all the potential that there is in the recovery community. Most people love to give of themselves, whether it's because of recovery or something else. (Volunteer)

We feel the Serenity Café is helping to add value to existing drug and alcohol services so that together we create better opportunities for people in recovery. White and Cloud (2008, p. 30) comments on the importance of linking treatment to community work, in recognition of "the inextricable link between personal, family, and community health … [recovery plans] include interventions to elevate family and community recovery capital and assertively link clients and families to other individuals, families, and community institutions rich in recovery capital." We have achieved this through increasing choice rather than simply increasing referrals—the passing of pro-forma between agencies, which their clients are meant to dutifully follow. This is an important distinction, because it seems to us that social networks cannot be artificially created—their value is that there is a bond formed between people based on mutual desire for it; what we are doing is bringing people together and creating opportunities in supportive conditions for this to take place. What we are also slowly developing is an alliance between a recovery community-led organization and professionalized organizations.

The Serenity Café has been incredibly fortunate to be developing at a time when a local treatment center, Lothian and Edinburgh Abstinence Program (LEAP), has become a center-stage initiative in Scotland. Its clinical lead has championed recovery and recognized the potential for the Serenity Café to bring a "multiplicative effect" (Rawson, 1994) for people leaving treatment, therefore generating new potential and enhancing all our contributions alongside the housing provision and educational provision of two other agencies. The alliance is helping Serenity Café to creep in from the sidelines and gain a seat at local planning partnerships through the LEAP clinical lead's patronage far more quickly than we could have achieved without this, and slowly, interest in our work is growing.

It is interesting that the emerging partnership between us has been organic and generated out of mutual interest rather than bureaucratic expediency, the driver for many other public and third sector partnerships. Our shared vision of creating recovery capital together is a form of collaborative advantage (Huxham, 1993) helping each organization achieve its own objectives better than we could alone but going further to create something additional which none of us could produce alone. But this is one factor in the development of the Serenity Café that is not necessarily replicable. Recovery champions who recognize the importance of positive community life for people in recovery need to be encouraged and nurtured and provided with evidence from practice to support their promotion of recovery.

Shared Outcomes

It appears then that one area where we can build strength together as partners and create a credible role for the Serenity Café is to find ways to be clear about the collaborative advantage and multiplicative effects we are creating together and to clarify the unique contributions each makes. Each organization negotiates a range of requirements from the contexts in which they operate: The treatment center is measured against waiting times, completion of the treatment program, and numbers leaving treatment intending to sustain abstinence from drug/alcohol, with follow-up measures associated with aftercare (although in many outcome studies, aftercare measurement has been weak); the housing provider is measured against transition into permanent tenancy, minimum arrears, and tenancy failure; the education provider is measured against attendance, qualifications gained, and transition into other destinations (college or employment). The Serenity Café, as yet uninhibited by funding that ties us to any specific policy intentions, is free to develop measures of success that can be oriented more clearly toward recovery. Like Valentine (as quoted in White, 2007, p. 90), we are not yet "bureaucratically bound" by rules, regulations, and paperwork. We are, as he says, "more free and unencumbered to sustain a focus on whatever it takes to support recovery," but we must not slip into the trap of gathering no evidence at all. Self-discipline is required in the absence of funders wielding the accountability whip. As White and Cloud (2008) point out, much of the work with people recovering from addiction is measured by what it reduces or subtracts (e.g., crime, substance use), not what it creates (quality of life, long-term recovery, belonging).

With our partners, we have agreed that the multiplicative effect we are creating together is recovery capital, a concept each is trying to make meaningful in the different policy and practice contexts in which we operate; and the Serenity Café has begun to explore with our volunteers and customers whether this is a meaningful concept in their world and their experience of our work.

Evolution and Evidence

The task now is to build on the framework as a tool for ongoing evaluation. Part of the challenge is to develop credible qualitative indicators in an environment in which we have noticed that medical/scientific measures, which can be statistically verified, are the dominant currency (notably avoiding at present the application of such rigorous measurement of long-term treatment outcomes).

We also face the challenge of trying to evaluate a range of processes involving *personal* development and empowerment, *collective* development and empowerment, and the growth of a community; trying to consider the linkages between these processes; and assessing our own contribution and those of other partners (multiplicative effect). It is complex and potentially messy. It would be tempting to opt for the crude and simple measures that many future funders might expect: number of jobs created, number of volunteer hours, number of customers and range of their activities, and income versus expenditure—all important, but falling somewhat short of the outcomes we believe are really achieved. As a small organization, our most pragmatic approach to this is to commit to faithfully recording the story of development as it unfolds. Evaluation is not just about accountability; it is about learning (Oakley, 2001), and it is important that we continually engage our volunteers and customers in this learning process, which in itself can become empowering. As Taylor (2000) cautions, "If not incorporated as an integral part of a conscious and concerted development practice, monitoring and evaluation are likely first to diminish and then undermine empowerment by reducing it to easily measurable elements that become a meaningless parody." Before we do (hopefully) become obliged to meet funders' needs for information that suits their bureaucratic systems, we do at least have some space now to experiment with our own methods of gathering evidence to support our contention that the development of recovery capital in individuals and the recovery community is a tangible outcome of the Serenity Café.

White and Cloud (2008, p. 30) again provide us with an organizing concept of community recovery capital with which our volunteers, customers, and partners easily identify:

- **active efforts to reduce addiction/recovery-related stigma**

   Stigma has a lot to do with it. So what Serenity has to do is educate that people in recovery are responsible and constructive members of society. (Café customer)

- **visible and diverse local recovery role models**

   The Serenity Café is a great place to learn about relationships. I need things in my life, my life isn't sorted, I need more than work in my life. It's good for me to be about people who are healthy in recovery. (Volunteer)

   In early recovery, I had a real fear of loneliness, of being alone, but to be with people, it needed to be people who shared the experience. (Café customer)

- **a full continuum of addiction treatment resources**

   I think that the Serenity Café would be a really good tool for the recovery belt. (Community survey)

   [Recovery] didn't happen in treatment; it happened when I started finding my place in life. (Volunteer)

- **recovery mutual aid resources that are accessible and diverse**

> It feels like being part of a community, not just a part of a meeting. Serenity Café is making recovery visible. (Volunteer)

- **local recovery community-support institutions**

> Lifesaver, proves there is an excellent night out without alcohol. (Customer feedback)

> Mainly I think Serenity Café is a great idea and good for the whole community; I feel it's like service and it builds my self-esteem. (Volunteer)

- **sources of sustained recovery support and early reintervention**

> To have a safe haven is essential to continued recovery. (Volunteer)

> Serenity Café is about how to live life outside meetings in the real world. (Café customer)

CONCLUSION

In summing up our work to develop the Serenity Café, we have provided an answer for ourselves to a question posed recently by a potential funder—why should a community development organization try to work in the addictions field? Our immediate answer had been: We are not working in the addictions field; we are working in the recovery field. Our exploration here of what we are doing and how it is working here confirms for us the value of community development and what this means in practice.

Community development is about addressing the underlying structural causes of social problems and their distressing consequences to reduce uncertainty and insecurity in people's lives. It encompasses attention to the material and spiritual needs of people, both their needs and their aspirations. It requires a democratic approach in which intentions, and the ways of achieving them, must be transparent and accountable to the people whose lives they touch (United Nations, 1995).

Serenity Café is helping people in recovery to take the wraps off recovery and bring it into the mainstream of city life. This has the potential to change the way we see recovery and the way we see treatment and the experience of addiction. The visibility of recovery is important in many ways. As Lerner (1990, p. 15) said, "The dominant culture is not threatened by sick people meeting together to get well." Volunteers themselves are certainly proud of their achievements, and through increasing solidarity, are gaining the skills and confidence to promote their views on recovery. We do not think we are simply empowering people in recovery as a subgroup that will remain on the margins of society, but we must be constantly vigilant about that risk. Some people in recovery have been concerned that we are trying to create an alternative community that will segregate people from the wider community, rather than create inclusion for people in recovery in our wider society. Our intention is to make the Serenity Café a place where people can build bridges to all kinds of future opportunities and where people of any background can learn more about recovery. At present, we do this by ensuring the Serenity Café is a place where families and friends feel welcome and enjoy the experience. We will endeavor to learn more about how/if the Serenity Café helps achieve inclusion as we develop.

What we have also confirmed for ourselves in this discussion of our work with the Serenity Café is the breadth of skills that have been required to support the initiative. This breadth is rarely available within specialized services, which tend to appoint people with a single specialism. We also enjoy the advantage of approaching the work without the baggage that weighs down many services in the drug and alcohol field. We are not proponents of one route to recovery, and we have had no need to categorize addiction by preferred substance, form of ingestion, risk assessment, or any criteria other than a person identifying a need to connect with others in recovery who are focusing on abstinence as their goal. We can be openly respectful of whatever means people find to achieve and sustain recovery, which in turn leads to opportunities for positive relationships with a wide range of other groups and organizations.

Many development initiatives are undertaken on the basis of the needs and deprivations of a particular group of people and still fail to recognize and build on the capacities of the individuals and groups involved. The literature on the growth of recovery communities, from which we have gained a great deal of strength and encouragement, is still at the stage of arguing for the relevance of this approach and for greater recognition of recovery capital. We hope this article adds to those articles' discussions of "why," with some insight into "how" recovery capital in individuals and recovery communities can develop.

I love my recovery. I love my life now. (Volunteer)

REFERENCES

Ashton, M. (2008, December/January). The new abstentionists. *Druglink, 23*(1), 1–16.

Bamber, S. (2009a). *Making sense of recovery identities*. Retrieved from http://www.theartoflifeitself.org

Bamber, S. (2009b, October). *Rethinking community: Addiction, recovery, and globalization*. Paper presented at the 12th International EWODOR Symposium, University of Stirling, Stirling, Scotland.

Bandura, A. (2006). Guide for creating self-efficacy scales. In F. Pajares & T. Urdan (Eds.), *Self-efficacy beliefs of adolescents* (pp. 307–337). Charlotte, NC: Information Age.

Best, D., Groshkova, T., & McTague, P. (2009). The politics of numbers: How target setting has blocked people's recovery from addiction. *Druglink, 24*(5), 16–17.

Burns, D., & Taylor, M. (1998). *Mutual aid and self-help coping strategies for excluded communities.* Bristol, UK: Policy Press and Joseph Rowntree Foundation.

Craig, T. (2008, September/October). Work in progress. *Druglink, 23*(5), 12–13.

Davis, M., & Jason, L. (2005). Sex differences in social support and self-efficacy within a recovery community. *American Journal of Community Psychology, 36*(3/4), 259–274.

Folgheraiter, F., & Pasani, A. (2009). Self-help groups and social capital: New directions in welfare policies? *Social Work Education, 28*(3), 253–267.

Gartner, A., & Reissman, F. (1979). *Self-help in the human services.* San Francisco, CA: Jossey Bass.

Huxham, C. (1993). Pursuing collaborative advantage. *Journal of the Operational Research Society, 44*(6), 599–611.

Kemp, R. (2009). Relating to the other: Truth and untruth in addiction. *European Journal of Psychotherapy and Counseling, 11*(4), 355–368.

Lerner, H. G. (1990). Problems for profit? *Women's Review of Books, 7*(7), 15–16.

McKeganey, M., & McIntosh, J. (2006, October). From addiction to work … a road to nowhere? *Drink and Drugs News*, p. 6–7.

McKeganey, N. (2008, March/April). The reaction. *Druglink, 28*(2), 18–19.

Neff, K. (2009). The role of self-compassion in development: A healthier way to relate to oneself. *Human Development, 52*, 211–214.

Oakley, P. (Ed.). (2001). *Evaluating empowerment—reviewing the concept in practice* (NGO Management and Policy Series No. 13). Oxford, UK: Intrac.

Paterson, S., Weaver, T., & Crawford, M. (2010). Drug service user groups: Only a partial solution to the problem of developing service user involvement. *Drugs: Education, Prevention, and Policy, 17*(1), 81–97.

Rawson, D. (1994). Models of interprofessional work: Likely theories and possibilities. In A. Leathard (Ed.), *Going interprofessional: Working together for health and welfare.* London, UK: Routledge.

Scottish Government. (2008a). *Changing Scotland's relationship with alcohol.* Edinburgh, Scotland: Author.

Scottish Government. (2008b). *The road to recovery: A new approach to tackling Scotland's drug problem.* Edinburgh, Scotland: Author.

Swanson, A. (2009, April 20). Thinking differently. Social enterprise special report. *Holyrood Magazine*, p. 8.

Taylor, J. (2000). So now they are going to measure empowerment! Community Development Resource Association. Retrieved from http://www.cdra.org.za/index.php?option=com_content&view=article&id=29%3Aso-now-they-are-going-to-measure-empowerment&Itemid=2

United Nations. (1995, March). *Copenhagen Declaration and Program of Action.* Paper presented at the World Summit for Social Development Copenhagen, Denmark.

Ward, D. (2000). Totem not token: Group work as a vehicle for user participation. In H. Kemshall & R. Littlechild (Eds.), *User involvement and participation in social care* (pp. 45–65). London, UK: Jessica Kingsley.

White, W. L. (2007). *Perspectives on systems transformation: How visionary leaders are shifting addiction treatment toward a recovery-oriented system of care.* Chicago, IL: Great Lakes Addiction Technology Transfer Center.

White, W., & Cloud, W. (2008). Recovery capital: A primer for addictions professionals. *Counselor, 9*(5), 22–27.

A Firsthand Account of Service User Groups in the United Kingdom: An Evaluation of Their Purpose, Effectiveness, and Place Within the Recovery Movement

MATTHEW KIDD

UK Recovery Academy, Glasgow, Scotland, United Kingdom

*This article will seek to understand and critique existing service user involvement through an analysis of existing forums. This analysis will explore the drivers that have led to the formation of such groups, explore the range and scope for involvement that these forums allow, and assess their effectiveness in relation to definitions of their purpose. The analysis will also seek to determine whether there are common factors that either progress or limit their ability to achieve their aims. On the basis of this evidence, and within the context of the growing recovery movement, the article will present a potential new model, or models, and definitions of service user involvement. It will also outline the development of one such model through an examination of **Uchooseit** (a peer support service in Tameside that is situated in the Northwest of England). In this way, the article will seek to stimulate debate over the vexed question of what service user involvement really means within the United Kingdom and how it may be defined in the future within the context of the recovery model.*

This essay will first look to define service user involvement before seeking to establish its purpose and place within treatment services, recovering communities, and the wider recovery movement. It will also look at the role of mutual aid and peer support and consider the role of peer support within user groups, recovery forums, and emerging recovery organizations.

In England, the National Health Service (NHS) offers what is referred to as "the mandatory drug service," in other words, prescribing treatments such as methadone, subutex, and naltrexone (all of which are used to treat opiate dependency). Other forms of treatment and support are open to tender, and any service that meets certain quality standards is open to bid for them. On the whole, the local drug and alcohol action teams (DAATs) are responsible for producing treatment plans that outline which services will be provided. There will often be an allocation in the plans and budgets of the DAAT for "service user involvement"—that is to say, current or former service users feeding back on the effectiveness of the services that are provided within the area. This essay will look to evaluate this model of service user involvement.

This model of service user involvement was established within a system of care that viewed addiction as a "chronic relapsing condition." The following design flaws with "acute care systems" in the United States have been identified:

> (They) inhibit client attraction, engagement, retention, and treatment completion, limit the scope and duration of professional services and re-covery support, provided during and following addiction treatment, and fail to assertively link individuals and families to indigenous communities of recovery. (White, 2009, p. 10)

This essay will seek to establish whether the same problems exist in the United Kingdom and will look at the role of user groups, recovery forums, and recovery organizations in addressing these problems.

In the United Kingdom, the work of Neil Small and Penny Rhodes has helped to define service user involvement within the NHS, and they have provided us with the following definition:

> Service user involvement can be loosely defined as the involvement or participation, on various levels, by people who access and use the ser-vices, in the design, planning and delivery of the services they receive. (Small & Rhodes, 2000, as cited in Plunkett, 2000, p. 15)

There are two or three significant problems when attempting to relate this definition to the experiences of those in recovery from drug and/or alcohol problems:

1. It presents people as if their main identity is through the consumption of services. People in recovery are unlikely to identify with this. It makes no reference to other aspects of an individual's life, their needs, or interests.
2. People in recovery may no longer access the services in question, and therefore, they are not in the best position to represent those who do.

3. Involvement in the design, planning, and delivery of services through means of a service user group can be, in reality, very limited.

In addition to defining service user involvement as a generic term, it is helpful to establish how the National Treatment Agency (NTA) views service user involvement. The **NTA** is a **NHS** special authority established to help improve the availability, capacity, and effectiveness of drug treatment in England. According to its Website:

> The NTA wants to build an equal partnership with treatment service users and drug users because we recognise that those in treatment and those who have identified a need for treatment have the right to become involved in activities that affect their health and well being. We respect the unique expertise and experiences of users and understand the health, esteem and other personal benefits that involvement can bring. (NTA, n.d.)

Again, this definition refers to people in treatment and drug users as though that is their main identity. It says nothing about promoting recovery and personal development and says little about issues such as empowerment and employability.

A possible implication of the NTA's definition of user involvement is that the NTA is looking for ways in which the "expertise" of service users can contribute to effective treatment. Although it is recognized that effective treatment should be an important part of any system of care, a recovery-focused system will look to meet a much more diverse range of needs. If all that someone in recovery can contribute is their experience of substance abuse and treatment, then these diverse needs are not being met. Service user involvement is restricted to how service users can contribute to a set model. It is also worth considering why people get involved in user groups. Is it a fair assumption to say that the main reason is because they want to see improvements in the treatment system?

EXPERIENCES OF TRADITIONAL USER GROUPS

In evaluating the effectiveness of user groups, it is important to look at the positives and negatives of the traditional model of the user group. I have attempted to do this through analysis of the views and experiences of those involved in service user groups. Limitations in terms of times and resources meant I could only access people from the Northwest of England. I spoke with around 20 members of service user groups past and present. I had initially hoped to conduct formal, structured interviews, but people had reservations about this. There appeared to be a reluctance to take part in formal research. These people did, however, agree to an informal discussion and gave their consent for me to use material from these discussions in this essay on the understanding that they would not be named or quoted directly. This is not an ideal way of gathering evidence, but it did provide people with the chance to relax and speak their mind. There is a good chance that this provided more honest answers than structured questionnaires and/or interviews would have done.

It is fair to say that some of the needs of those involved in user groups were being met; some had been involved in service user groups for well over 12 months, which alone suggests that they must serve something of a social support function.

However, there appeared to be many limitations placed on those who were involved with traditional user groups. Too many activities seemed to revolve around representation. That is not to say that there is not merit in representation; it does serve a purpose. Of those I spoke with, the vast majority felt that service managers and commissioners[1] respected their opinions and were fairly receptive to new ideas. In turn, this often resulted in an increase in confidence and self-esteem. There were also benefits in terms of building a network: Almost all the service users I spoke with stated that they made useful contacts during their time as a member of a service user group. When I asked why people had joined user groups, the predominant response was that they were looking for something to fill their time now that they had stopped using or drinking. Only two of those with whom I spoke mentioned wishing to improve services. There was a common theme of "wanting to put something back," but this was more driven by a desire to provide peer/social support than a need to right the wrongs of the treatment services.

There was a great deal of frustration about the amount of time it took to get new ideas off the ground. My personal experience corresponds with this. I felt that many of the meetings I attended held little or no relevance to me and that my presence was little more than a box-ticking exercise. Although I do feel that I managed to earn the respect of the majority of those present at such meetings, I was left a little disillusioned about the lack of progress with the issues I raised. Indeed this was a common theme: There was a huge gap between acknowledging things were not working and putting them right. Constraints on time and budgets were possibly bigger reasons for this than not realizing the value of what service users (or former service users) were saying.

Attending strategic meetings and events, alongside the occasional drop-in, seemed to account for the vast majority of activities user groups were involved in. People's time and input were limited during strategic meetings, and many people commented on being extremely bored in many of the more formal meetings. The main focus of the drop-ins was to provide refreshments and "a friendly ear" to people accessing drug and alcohol treatment. Some of the people I spoke with expressed a desire to run these out of the treatment setting, as it was rarely conducive to open discussion.

My opinion as to the reason for the narrow scope of the service user groups is that it is the product of a risk-averse system. There appears to be a great deal of fear surrounding things that may go wrong with peer-led groups and activities. There was also a feeling among some of those I spoke with that some members of staff failed to take them seriously and that some health care professionals saw little merit in any activity not facilitated by "a trained professional." It is possible that this trend is a local one; as I only spoke with people from Tameside, Stockport, and Oldham, United Kingdom (all within a 10 mile radius on the outskirts of Greater Manchester), this may well be the case.

With the right training and support in place, the majority of those with whom I spoke felt that service user groups could act as a platform to education, training, and voluntary work. This was also a view shared by many members of staff. This function would appear to be one of the long-term merits of such groups. As I stated earlier, their predominant reason for joining a user group was to spend time more productively. The majority also said that they would like something to show for their time and commitment.

Opportunities to progress for those involved in such groups tend to be created through networking and improvements in confidence, self-esteem, motivation, and determination. There is very little in the way of training provided. There may well be a place for a course that serves the purpose of "learning to learn" alongside other activities that provide the supervision and support needed to progress in education, training, and employment.

Service user groups tend to be independent of any particular service provider, and they tend to be funded directly by the DAAT.[2] This is for the purposes of accountability: If the user groups were dependent on a particular service for funding, then there may be an expectation that they are not overly critical of said service. The DAATs often employ a service user development worker or service user group coordinator to act in an advisory capacity. Among those with whom I spoke, there were mixed feelings about someone being employed in such a post. The development worker tends to work as a "middle man" liaising between the user group and the service providers. The development worker role also involved assisting with the organizational side of things. It appeared to some that there was a conflict of interests here. The person in this role was supposed to empower the service users to take more responsibility, but if they afforded them too much, then they might become redundant. Indeed, one person who I spoke with said that their relationship with their development worker started off very positively before reaching a "brick wall" stage. At this stage, they began to feel resentful of the development worker and felt they were being actively discouraged from taking on more responsibility.

The flip side to this is that some of those with whom I spoke felt there was a need for the development worker in terms of orientation and support, particularly in the early stages. Although there may well be a need for someone to provide this support, it appears to me that there is a conflict of interests if someone's role consists solely of providing this support. As people progress, there is a consensus that they should be allowed to take more ownership and responsibility. Indeed, there is a strong argument to suggest that a more experienced member of the user group could provide this support.

Having looked at the merits of the traditional model of the user group, it is important to look at how we can maintain any support structures while also tackling the problems with many of the traditional user groups. It would also be useful to look at the role of peer support in relation to the mandatory services. To move toward recovery-oriented integrated systems, relations between mandatory services, the third sector, and user groups need to be more clearly established and defined. In the current climate, it is highly unlikely that DAATs will spend a large amount of money to revolutionize the mandatory services.[3] It is even more unlikely that they will employ more key workers to provide a more individualized, person-centered approach (i.e., workers spending more time with their clients to respond to all of their needs). Bearing this in mind, the roles of volunteers and peer supporters become crucial.

EMERGING MODELS OF USER INVOLVEMENT

So how does this work in practice? To establish this, I will look at three emerging recovery organizations: *Uchooseit* in Tameside, the *Basement Project* in Halifax, and *Those on the Margins of a Society* (*THOMAS*) in Blackburn (all of which are in the North of England). I will then look to establish the shared success factors. I will also look to establish the benefits of links with mutual aid groups such as Alcoholics Anonymous (AA), Narcotics Anonymous (NA), and Self-Management and Recovery Training (SMART) recovery.

Uchooseit in Tameside is a good example of a peer-led organization with activities and ethos that cater to the diverse need of service users and people in recovery. In March 2009, members of a traditional service group drafted a proposal for a peer-led signposting service (*Uchooseit*). This service would build strong links with agencies that deal with issues such as housing, debt, employment, and education and would act as a community resource that would assist people in addressing their practical needs. Another key function of the service would be to provide training and volunteering opportunities for people in recovery.

It soon became apparent that **Uchooseit** was the right idea at the right time. Those involved knew from their own personal experience how much of a need there was for a service like this in Tameside. Indeed, frustration with the gaps in service provision was one of the driving forces in **Uchooseit**'s inception. The appetite for an organization such as this was also enhanced by the emergence of the recovery movement. The importance of recovery capital was becoming more apparent.[4]

Uchooseit is now established as a community interest company (CIC)[5] and offers a wide range of activities including breakfast and lunchtime meals for the homeless and people in poverty, a women's group, sports and recreational activities, and a peer-mentoring scheme. There are currently more than 20 volunteers from a wide range of backgrounds who are engaged with **Uchooseit.** It is important to note that one of the key functions of the volunteering program is to provide training, supervision, and support, which was notable because its absence in the traditional user groups. As a direct result of being involved in **Uchooseit**, people have gained qualifications such as NVQ (National Vocational Qualification) in advice and guidance and a whole host of experience, which can not only improve an individual's employability but improve internal recovery capital in the form of improved confidence and self-esteem.

The **Basement Project** in Halifax is another example. Indeed, this organization influenced **Uchooseit** a great deal. One of the key strengths of the **Basement Project** is just how different it is to anything that existed in Halifax beforehand. The project's Web site gives an accurate description: "The project has evolved primarily as a response to gaps in service delivery and now enjoys a positive reputation for effective and flexible service delivery through partnership working at the cutting edge of the changing direction in substance misuse treatment."

The **Basement Project** provides a user-led drop-in breakfast club, which allows engagement with the most hard-to-reach clients. They have a volunteer training program in which they recruit many of their (former) service users, some of whom are now employed by the **Basement Project**. Many volunteers who complete the recovery program now work as peer mentors to others coming through recovery.

THOMAS in Blackburn has a similar ethos to **Uchooseit** and the **Basement Project**. The organization's CEO, James McCartney (n.d.), calls for "a greater focus on holistic development and a move away from the domination of the clinical concept of treatment." He adds: "We need to elevate the concept of human development at the forefront of strategic thinking."

THOMAS provides the following services: 26-week residential rehabilitation program, support for ex-offenders, community-based support, employment opportunities for ex-offenders and former drug users, mentoring ex-offenders on release from prison, drama workshops on drugs for schools and colleges, and a drop-in center that feeds up to 70 people per day.

Organizations such as this focus on what they can offer to the individuals involved, and how they can address some of the gaps in service provision. This is opposed to the traditional model of the service user group, which looked to inform the mandatory services of the needs of service users but did little in the way of responding to these needs in their own right. ***Uchooseit***, ***The Basement Project***, ***THOMAS,*** and other like-minded services are helping to establish a developing model of service user involvement, one in which the experiences of those in recovery play an integral part. In this developing model, service users and people in recovery are treated with due respect, and their opinions and experiences are equally valid to those of the service managers. The current model may consult service users on issues around treatment, but these emerging recovery organizations can truly lay claim to involving service users in planning, design, and delivery.

Emerging recovery organizations act as a community resource and can respond to the needs of people throughout their recovery journey. They establish strong links with other services within the community and promote recovery, while helping to establish that people recovering from drug and alcohol problems have a lot to offer.

THE ROLE OF MUTUAL AID

Emerging recovery organizations promote the concept of people in recovery helping one another. This concept is, however, nothing new. Mutual aid groups have long been operating on this premise. Keith Humphries summarizes common components of mutual aid groups in his book *Circles of Recovery* (as cited in McCartney, 2010). Members share the same problem or status, groups are organized and facilitated by members themselves, experiential knowledge is the basis of expertise, all members are both "helpers" and "helpees," and no fees are charged, save for pass-the-hat contributions (McCartney, 2010).

The most famous mutual aid group is AA, which defines itself thusly:

> Alcoholics Anonymous is a fellowship of men and women who share their experience, strength and hope with each other that may solve their common problem and help others recover from alcoholism. The only requirement for membership is a desire to stop drinking. There are no dues or fees for AA membership; we are self-supporting through our own contributions. (Alcoholics Anonymous, 2010)

There are many other "Anonymous" groups such as NA and Cocaine Anonymous, which operate on more or less the same premise (just substitute alcoholism for drug addiction, cocaine addiction, etc.).

SMART recovery is a fairly recent addition to the family of mutual aid groups and emerged in the United States in 1994 (McCartney, 2010). The main way in which it differs from the "Anonymous" groups is that it does not follow a spiritual, 12-step program. Instead, SMART recovery promotes a four-point recovery program:

1. Enhancing and maintaining motivation to abstain;
2. Coping with urges;
3. Problem solving; and
4. Lifestyle balance.

In the United Kingdom, SMART is mainly delivered by trained volunteers, preferably people who have "gained independence from addictive behaviour through participation in SMART recovery" (SMART Recovery UK, 2010). SMART recovery in the United Kingdom believes that "individuals who have been successful in gaining independence from addictive behaviours appear to have made changes in all four areas we teach about" (SMART Recovery UK, 2010).

The following have been identified (among others) as key functions of peer-led, or peer-based, services: to identify resources that support recovery, assertive linkage to communities of recovery, and responding to needs (White, 2009, p. 28).

If user groups and peer-led organizations are to act as a community resource, then it is in their best interests to establish and maintain strong links with mutual aid groups. They should be in a position to inform others as to how to access them and what to expect from them. It is important that individuals are kept informed about all their options and that they are given real choice and variety in the services and activities they may wish to access. Indeed, one of the key functions of peer-led organization and user groups is to act as an "honest broker," with no hidden agendas or preferences. The job of the peer-led service is merely to identify the resources and link people to them, not to form judgments on them or promote one over another.

> There are many roads to recovery and each one is individual. However, many travel the roads together, at least for a period, and for many their paths will intersect in mutual aid groups. (McCartney, 2010)

CONCLUSION

So far in this essay, we have looked at how the traditional model of service user involvement sat within a system that was dominated by "the clinical concept of treatment" and how it could be said that service users were consulted, but not necessarily involved in, service delivery. We also established some of the benefits of the traditional model of the user group, such as the importance of networking and building a support structure.

We moved on to view the role of service user involvement within emerging recovery organizations and identified some key strengths and shared success factors of such organizations. We then looked at the role of mutual aid groups within the recovery movement.

We are hopefully now in a position to answer some key questions. Is there a new or developing model of service user involvement, and is it more effective than the old one?

There is growing evidence to suggest that there is a developing model of service user involvement as evidenced by the emerging recovery organizations listed in this essay. Is it more effective? Well, it is almost impossible to answer this question without bias on the limited evidence we have to date. What I can say with a fair amount of confidence is that this developing model of service user involvement is more recovery focused in that it provides more opportunity to build recovery capital. This developing model also caters more toward individual needs and personal development.

Uchooseit has also successfully married the need to feedback on issues relating to the effectiveness of treatment and support services in a way in which the person in recovery is viewed as the expert. This has been done in two ways. Firstly, instead of "token service user representation," *Uchooseit* now offers training and support to people who wish to act as an "expert patient." Expert patients have sat on tendering panels,[6] with exactly the same roles and responsibilities as commissioners, service managers, and general practitioners. The second way is through recovery workshops in which people in recovery prepare a 10-minute talk on their experiences of treatment, support, and recovery services. They highlight what worked well and what did not work so well before opening up a group discussion in which professionals from Tier 2 and Tier 3[7] services ask questions to gain a greater understanding of what it takes for someone to achieve and maintain recovery. These activities do truly create an equal partnership, and the *Uchooseit* volunteers who have taken part so far said they felt their opinions were truly valued and that this had a positive effect on their confidence and esteem.

People who are in recovery, or are seeking recovery, and are involved with emerging recovery organizations such as *Uchooseit*, *The Basement Project* and *THOMAS* have genuine choice. Their involvement is not defined by the fact that they have used services.

Is the recovery movement at odds with the NHS and other statutory services?[8] There is no short answer to this question; in fact, this question could be an essay in itself. If we identify that one of the key principles of recovery is that it is "not in opposition to harm-reduction programmes" (SAMHA, 2009), then we can establish that it need not be. There is a role for user groups and peer-led organizations in promoting recovery and culture change, within both drug and alcohol services and the wider community. There will continue to be constraints on those who work in statutory services, but with more clearly defined and established links with peer groups and the third sector, we can ensure that this does not come at the cost of those in, or working toward, recovery. This article has outlined some of the ways in which the tensions between health care "professionals" and "service users" can be eased; I speak in particular of the recovery workshops that **Uchooseit** delivered alongside the Tameside third sector coalition. Through these workshops, NHS workers identified the need to "make recovery more visible," "create more volunteering opportunities for people in recovery," and "address stigma and fear." The NTA speaks of an "equal partnership" but is easy to make a case to say that the established structure of service user involvement does not provide this.

The developing model of user involvement perhaps goes even further than the suggestion of "equal partnership" and identifies the (former) service user as the expert. The conversations I have had with people in preparing for this essay have also identified that being referred to as a "service user" or even "service user representative" can have a negative effect on self-esteem. It is worth asking the question of whether referring to people who work in drug and alcohol services as "professionals" or "workers" and to members of service user groups as "service users" is conducive to an equal partnership. In the developing model, people do not have to identify themselves in such a way and can refer to themselves in a way which does not refer to the fact that they are or were "in treatment."

It seems crucial to me to support the development of emerging recovery organizations to ensure that they become a valued part of every system of care. As we see the emergence of many new recovery forums,[9] it is important that they do not sit in isolation from the other treatment and support services. We must recognize the value of people in recovery and peer supporters in building social supports and expanding recovery capital. It is only through recovery forums and peer-led services that people in recovery can become visible. Once these people become visible recovery champions, they can help people to believe that recovery is not only possible but desirable. I refer to both people who provide and people who receive treatment and support services.

The experiences of those involved in user groups in the Northwest of England seem to indicate that traditional user forums struggled to find a clear and defined role within local systems of care. Their role was primarily to represent the views of service users, but this appears to have limited effect. By contrast, the recovery workshops I have referred to in this essay immediately helped to address stigma and shape the attitudes and beliefs of local health care professionals. It would be perhaps unfair to state that the traditional model of user involvement has entirely failed in its aim to "respect the unique expertise and experiences of users and understand the health, esteem and other personal benefits that involvement can bring" (NTA, n.d.), but it would be fair to say that the established structure has weaknesses that need to be addressed.

NOTES

1. Commissioners tend to work for DAATs, and their role is to decide which services need to be commissioned in the local area.

2. DAATs are drug and alcohol action teams, and their role is to produce treatment/recovery plans, allocate budgets, and monitor performance of local services. Scotland and Wales do not have DAATs, as they are not affiliated with the NTA.

3. Prescribing treatment is referred to as a "mandatory service." Certain services related to the criminal justice system are also referred to as "mandatory services."

4. Recovery capital is the internal and external "assets" that make an individual more likely to succeed in their recovery. Internal assets include things such as life satisfaction, confidence, and esteem; external assets include things such as secure housing.

5. CICs are similar to charities but differ in that they are allowed to generate a profit as long as they use this profit to the benefit of the community.

6. A tendering panel evaluates proposals to provide a specified service that has "gone to tender."

7. Tier 2 services are open-access services, which provide advice and support. Tier 3 services are more clinical services, which provide prescribing services and structured one-to-one appointments.

8. Statutory services are services that every area in England is obligated to provide. Other than prescribing services, this mainly refers to the criminal justice system and drug rehabilitation requirements.

9. A recovery forum is an alternative to a service user group. The key difference is that recovery forums look to cater specifically to the needs of people in recovery as opposed to those still accessing treatment services.

REFERENCES

Alcoholics Anonymous. (2010). *Alcoholics Anonymous Great Britain*. Retrieved from http://www.alcoholics-anonymous.org.uk/

McCartney, D. (2010). Mutual aid in the UK. [Weblog post]. Retrieved from http://wiredin.org.uk/blogs/entry/7453/mutual-aid-in-the-uk

McCartney, J. (n.d.). *The Challenge for the Public Sector*. THOMAS. Retrieved from http://www.thomasonline.org.uk/third_sector.htm

NTA. (n.d.). *Service users, families, and carers: How can service users or carers get involved?* National Treatment Agency for Substance Misuse. Retrieved from http://www.nta.nhs.uk/Who-service-involved.aspx

Plunkett, M. (2008). *User involvement in alcohol services: Myth or reality?: A literature review*. Glasgow, Scotland: MP Consultancy and NHS Health Scotland.

SAMHA. (2009). 12 guiding principles of recovery. *SAMHA News, 17*(5). Retrieved from http://www.samhsa.gov/samhsanewsletter/Volume_17_Number_5/GuidingPrinciples.aspx

SMART Recovery UK. (2010). About SMART Recovery. Retrieved from http://www.smartrecovery.org.uk/about

White, W. (2009). Peer-based addiction recovery support: History, theory, practice and scientific evaluation. *Counselor, 10*(5), 54–59.

A Tale of the Spontaneous Emergence of a Recovery Group and the Characteristics That Are Making It Thrive: Exploring the Politics and Knowledge of Recovery

WULF LIVINGSTON

Social Work Department, Glyndwr University, Wrecsam, United Kingdom

MATT BAKER

Psychology Student, Open University, Milton Keynes, United Kingdom

SIDNEY JOBBER and BOB ATKINS

DARE, Colwyn Bay, United Kingdom

This article details the history of an informal recovery-orientated mountaineering group based in North Wales. Although by definition a study rather than a research project, it nonetheless seeks to use the principles of narrative research as a means of evidencing the existence of activity-orientated recovery groups, illustrating their diversity and exploring the issues of knowledge and power that arguably construct and restrict recovery agendas. What will be presented is both a successful and typical mutual aid story (all be it in a more unusual context), springing from accidental beginnings but then progressing through initial bonding and forming to the long-term realization and maintenance of support. It will explore why belief in others, acts of giving and sharing, access to resources, and the taking of risks are fundamental ontological considerations for the recovery movement. Further, a tale of philosophies, knowledge, ownership, power, and recognition of achievement will provide evidence of what in other sectors would be called successful treatment outcomes but in reality actually offer challenges to rethink traditional treatment approaches and embrace a wider recovery-orientated perspective. This exploration of the evolution of

a functional and successful participant-owned recovery group will
be linked to conceptual models of recovery and change.

The story begins with a conversation between Adam,[1] a recovering drug user in the "treatment" system, and Brian, a worker providing a specifically commissioned intervention designed to help Adam get into work. Brian asks Adam a standard motivational interviewing question about his barriers and key anxieties, something along the lines of: "Tell me, what is the one thing you would really like to change?" Brian replies, "I need to and cannot find a qualified mountain guide—a group of us in rehab want to do this big mountain walk for charity." In most discourses, Brian's reply would be a sympathetic but ultimately unhelpful platitude ("I'm sorry to hear that, but would you like help with your CV/a cup of coffee/a leaflet about self employment?"). In our story, fate plays a role and the answer becomes, "I'm a qualified mountain guide—do you want a hand?"

What follows is a 5-year story detailing the birth, growth, and maturing of Drug and Alcohol Recovery Expeditions (DARE), a recovery-orientated mountaineering group, and more importantly—in a world where strategies, organizations, and ideas come and go—its continued existence. We will use this story to show how recovery and recovery groups exist in diverse formats often independent of (and arguably in contradiction to) strategically created and nationally managed programs. This will be done with reference to other recovery-orientated groups in the same wider North Wales community. Through this process of storytelling, we intend to explore certain issues surrounding the politics of recovery and associated notions of ownership of knowledge. By this, we mean that the history of DARE contains critical moments in terms of direction, response of others, mutual support, ownership, and unconditional positive regard—in essence, points which can be generalized and applied to other successful recovery movements. In doing so, and by being explicit in not claiming this as directly replicable research, we have nonetheless used some of the principles of case study design and narrative discourse: specifically, an analysis of a unique and boundaried system, the giving of attributable meaning to tales, and our informed theoretical notions of propositions about recovery groups (Yin, 2009). This approach reflects an acknowledgment of our interest in the highly contextual present perspective and any associated lack of control over wider events and variables (Yin).

Returning to our core story, Adam says to Brian, "That's fantastic, but how much is it going to cost? All the other guides want so much money it will make fundraising for charity pointless." Brian replies that he will do it for nothing. This giving of time by Brian without the expectation that it forms part of a work role is hugely important, associated as it is with notions of giving, equality, unity, and community. Perhaps sadly (but seemingly inevitably) issues of control and resources remain at the heart of the politics associated with recovery: This concept of "going the extra mile" will unfold through this account.

When Brian inquires further, it transpires that Adam and his peers from the rehabilitation unit want to undertake a walk known as the "15 Peaks" (e.g., Clayton & Turnbull, 2003). This involves a continuous expedition that attempts to cross the fifteen 3,000-foot (1,000 meter) plus mountains of North Wales in less than 24 hours. At around 30 miles, this challenge is significantly longer than a marathon and includes more than 13,000 feet of climbing (equivalent to halfway up Everest). Brian is inspired by this ambition and believes in the rehab folks' ability to do it. This belief in others' desire/competency to achieve and change (the "can do" assumption) is very much at the heart of this story and equally pertinent (sometimes for the wrong reasons) to the politics of recovery in general. Thus, Brian says to Adam: "Go and talk to Chris. I am sure he will help, walk with you, and he can probably access a bit of money for minibuses and the like." Chris also responded positively and became one of the long-term supporters of the group.

The next few months saw a small group (six to eight people, plus Adam and Chris) meet in the hills on a regular basis, communicating, bonding, and training. Despite being on a mountainside and not in a room full of appropriate agency furnishings, this followed the typical group-work evolution and all the stages of Tuckerman's *forming, norming, storming, and performing* model were to be seen (Douglas, 1993). The event itself was planned and attempted and resulted in 20 odd miles of walking over eight mountains in 18 hours. Three months later, 14 computers were exported to a school in South Africa that previously had none. The folks who had walked together found that they liked it so much that they wanted to continue to do it thereafter: An informal walking group had thus evolved.

This group has now been meeting monthly for 5 years. More than 100 members have come and gone; an ever-increasing core contingent have come and stayed. These "long termers" have built up a foundation of experience and skills (mountain and life related) that are shared with new participants. Many different summits have been visited; numerous personal goals have been achieved. Folks who did not think they could did. A second attempt was made at the 15 Peaks—more people took part, more support was in place, and more money was raised. At the third attempt, 8 members of the group walked for 27 hours through two sunrises and several moments of sugar-depleted mountain madness before limping off the final peak in a sun burnt but triumphant haze. More recently, the group became constituted as DARE and is working toward affiliation with the British Mountaineering Council. The interests of specific members have steered it gently into scrambling, caving, and climbing. It has a small supply of equipment to support new members but continues to exist largely on the basis of cooperative goodwill. It is also responsible in part for the creation by two of its members of a pilot project called Evolve Outdoors, which is providing therapeutic outdoor education-based interventions to those with substance misuse and offending history.

In terms of making a more informed understanding of this success, we are left with a number of questions and themes to explore: How has this happened? What makes it work? Can we evidence that this has helped members' recovery? Is it recovery in action? Why is this sort of thing not part of the mainstream? How is this different? We feel that exploration of these questions and the answers thus provided will offer us a legitimate and functional description of a recovery group in action. We further believe that it sheds some light on the politics and knowledge associated with recovery agendas.

CHARACTERISTICS FOR SURVIVAL

Turning to the first theme of these questions, that of beginnings and sustained survival, an explanation can perhaps be found by isolating one scenario from the tale as a whole. Imagine this scene from one of the regular walks: Twelve folks are sitting on the lower slopes of a hill having descended from the summit, admiring glorious views, basking in the presence of good company and the warm glow of achievement. They are asked if the group should become more formal and be officially registered, whether they are concerned about risk assessments, insurance, and constitutional form. The group rejects these considerations bluntly and unanimously, citing the giving, the sharing, the mutuality of support, and ownership as the power of the group. It is clear in this response (and in conversation at every monthly meeting) that they see the group in terms of a relationship of equals, a group of people on a shared literal and metaphorical journey. It is this, in its simplicity, that makes DARE what it is and underpins the fact that it continues to exist and work effectively for its members. The overtones of some of the core fundamentals of the mutual aid movements are evident within this and (we believe) enable us to claim this as an example of a recovery group in action.

The group evolved naturally from good fortune and an almost accidental meeting: This conversation between Adam and Brian might not have happened on another day or in another place and could not have happened if another worker was on shift. Such serendipitous moments can be identified in the evolution of other local groups, and their importance cannot be underestimated; they have, for instance, been cited as crucial to the history of one of the biggest recovery movements: Alcoholics Anonymous (Kurtz, 1991). This same North Wales "recovery community" has also spawned a vibrant performance and music group, an award-winning bakery, an on-line radio station, and the aforementioned Evolve. It is therefore possible that something similar might have occurred eventually through some similar propinquity. However, these other North Wales groups have all emerged largely as a consequence of accidental meetings between like-minded individuals committed to spending time and energy on what they feel is important, rather than being established via some strategically commissioned process. Crucial to the argument within this article is the idea that you cannot commission recovery but must seek instead to foster environments in which it can thrive. Ultimately, recovery movements are born from the desire of a collection of individuals to support each other through change, rather than be supported through change by someone not appearing to undertake the same change themselves. So a walking group for clients of an alcohol or drug service could be commissioned, but it would not be owned by the recovering folks nor feel the same to them or achieve the same collective and personal outcomes. The idea that the group reactively evolves according to the desires and motivations of its participants, rather than through application of a prescriptive "how to" manual, is why this article seeks simply to explore the characteristics and factors that facilitate this and deliberately avoids offering a step-by-step guide to replication—an approach that would be contradictory to our understanding of spontaneous recovery groups.

Thus, although the DARE group has three core members (Brian, Chris, and another, David) who might not necessarily be described as on the same alcohol and drug recovery journey as the group as a whole and who have had day jobs as "social care" employees, it is owned and run by the folks (White, 2007). Any role Brian, Chris, and David have had and do have has been consistent with that of the *acompanamiento*, as described by Whitmore and McGee (2001; cited in Bradbury & Reason, 2003). In this sense, the role of the "outsider" or "worker" (if recognized as such—Brian, Chris, and David have not always been viewed in this light by all the walkers) is to accompany the existing process of the group's growth and therefore to participate in an environment that creates mutual support, trust, common commitment, and solidarity (Bradbury & Reason). The DARE group encapsulates this commitment to collective ownership through voluntary participation; no one is out on the hills as a compulsory consequence of any part of another program they are involved in. This includes Brian, Chris, and David, who participate in their own and not during work time and who—perhaps crucially—regard participation as a leisure activity and pleasure.

Further underpinning this group-led and self-dependent identity is the fact that DARE is largely financially independent. It has in its 5-year history received three very small sums of external financial support (less than £3,000), certainly totaling less than that required by most community projects. Early in DARE's history, a statutory sector agency donated enough money to buy six basic sets of boots and waterproofs. More recently, the now formal committee was successful in acquiring a grant of a similar size from a national charity to purchase climbing and camping equipment. Occasionally throughout the group's history, it has had donations covering the cost of minibus hire from a local government organization. Although it has enhanced the experience of the group and its individuals, this money has not been essential. During regular monthly meetings, it is the membership that put their hands in their pockets to ensure the group functions. This is done through both the lending and giving of spare equipment to those without and through the use of private cars and petrol to meet the travelling costs of getting to and from the mountains.

Arguably, this equates to a normative financial journey for small non-statutory organizations and recovery groups, an existence without funding on the margins of the mainstream. The important point to make here is that access to resources has long been and remains a complex power issue for the recovery movement. The suggestion that spending money on mountains (or any alternative approach) rather than methadone makes humanitarian and economic sense horrifies some more traditional commentators. A quick trawl of the Daily Mail Web site illustrates this point by returning dozens of stories expressing outrage at the liberal treatment of drug addicts apparently given free holidays/drugs/activities/iPods/football tickets, etc. (Daily Mail, 2010). This echoes the vast challenges faced by all abstinence-based, non-medical, service user-led approaches that continue to operate in spite of the dominance of the professionally controlled, medically orientated provisions.

Membership of and participation in DARE is—perhaps obviously and certainly essentially—entirely free. The group, while centered on a core set of drug and alcohol users, does not hold "us and them" boundaries; it welcomes all comers. Walks frequently include wider family and community members, their dogs, and (occasionally) their daughters. In the complex construction of power and ownership, what therefore takes places is not a process that belongs to official others but to the folks themselves. Ownership of DARE and wider recovery movements is, however, about much more than membership and monies; it is a broader issue that runs all the way to the core of what recovery is and what can and cannot be described as recovery groups. The DARE members define both the group and their own difficulties; they consequently identify the solutions that allow them to realize the ambition of being in and on the hills, a process which parallels their wider journey.

Ownership of these journeys is both literal and metaphorical. Most walks are preceded by conversations about what to do and where to go, and always start with a shared moment of route construction in the car park. It is the DARE members who choose to undertake a DARE journey, not a detached group of professionals. Likewise, it is the DARE members who choose to place their faith in a given individual or group, in a situation where participants are equally reciprocal as givers and takers and where the primary purpose (and resulting beneficiaries) of the effort of the group are the group members themselves. Folks have a choice and literally vote with their feet.

This analogous representation is so crucial to the distinction between the recovery movement and the more traditional walking group and treatment agency approaches, where the staff members from the outdoor pursuits center have already determined which mountain will be walked, or where drug workers have already mapped out the direction and style of a clients' treatment plan. We suspect it would be hard to describe UK mainstream treatment services in the terms of DARE—a fact that enables us to identify and define what might be more accurately referred to as a recovery group (Bamber, 2010) in opposition to this statutory model. All participants bring something to DARE, and all receive something in return.

Belief in other people, other possibilities, and other ways of undertaking journeys is fundamental to the philosophy of the group. Due to the formal and informal interactions of the members prior to any given walk, most folks take part for the first time with a belief that they can do it already installed in them. Thus, the group performs "motivational interviewing" with potential new members, while standing on the street corner, over a cup of tea, or while sharing some other moment of understanding. It does not occur to anyone in the group that someone cannot get up a mountain (at least, not until they have been halfway up one for 3 hours contemplating the meaning of physical reality). We would, however, emphasize that the group has sufficient expertise to respond safely to the occasional sudden changes of plan that result from this structure and that this approach arguably initiates a form of positive labeling (e.g., Becker, 1963) that on balance tends to breed success.

Crucial to the supporting of belief is the initial response from agency, worker, support service, or peer. This tale began with a moment of trust, a crucial power issue. Fortunately, Brian did not even question Adam's belief in his and others' ability to do the walk but rather acknowledged their need as they described it. Brian believed in Adam and the others' ability to achieve. The initial motivational discourse between folks within the group and potential new members is never one of a restrictive, "No, you can't/Not yet" type, but one of a "Yes, you can" nature. Clients engaged in the narrower treatment system often experience a worker holding on to or reigning in their aspirations, the consequence of misinterpreted perspectives on what is or is not achievable, and the tendency of the worker to base expectation of an individual's likely success on their experience of previous average (often low) outcomes. Frequently, what restricts these dialogues between workers in treatment systems and clients is a failure to hear the drinker or drug user's desired starting and finishing points, rather than the agency's desired provision criteria and commissioned outcomes.

Simplistically put, DARE exists and continues to do so because people want it to. They have an investment in and ownership of a group, which, as we will explore, then gives them something valued back.

IS THIS A RECOVERY GROUP?

In understanding and identifying DARE as a recovery group, it is important to be able to identify it in terms of accepted collective definitions of both the term "recovery" and the term "group." This is doubly important at the current time, as the term "recovery" is increasingly claimed, used, and contested by agencies and informal groups, a fact set against the backdrop of a possible paradigm shift in alcohol and other drug-related strategies, commissioning, services, and treatment provision (The Scottish Government, 2008; White, 2007, 2009).[2]

It is probably easier (and less contentious) to define a group than it is to define recovery. It can further (obviously) be assumed that a recovery group will probably need to meet definitions of both these elements. Thus, a group can be defined simply as:

> ... two or more persons who are interacting with one another in such a manner that each person influences and is influenced by each other person. (Shaw, 1976)

White (2007) explores the difficulty of defining recovery before adopting a definition of it as:

> ... the experience (a process and a sustained status) through which individuals, families, and communities impacted by severe alcohol and other drug (AOD) problems [utilize] internal and external resources to voluntarily resolve these problems, heal the wounds inflicted by AOD related problems, actively manage their continued vulnerability to such problems, and develop a healthy, productive, and meaningful life. (p. 236)

This has in recent years been increasingly fore-shortened to something like:

> ... voluntary recovery maintained lifestyle [characterized] by sobriety, personal health and citizenship ... (McLellan, 2010)

In DARE, it is possible to see both a group (folks influencing each other through interaction with one another) and recovery that is supporting the active management of (their own and others) vulnerability through sustainable healthy and meaningful lifestyles. This utilizes some internal (personal) and external (group, community, and environmental) resources to enable folks to successfully explore and begin to resolve some of the formative causes and consequences of their drink and drug use.

The notion of the journey taken in DARE is of course both actual and metaphorical, where the group undertakes real physical journeys, has a collective tale of getting from A to B, and plays a role in individuals' own personal recovery tales. This symbolism is even more evident in the notion of people climbing mountains. Thus, time spent walking or in the mountains is always about more than just the notion of physically getting to the summit. For the most part, the acquired physical achievement is secondary to two other outcomes: that of overcoming personal mental challenges and that of being part of a group on a collective experiential journey. The group adopts a very simple philosophy when out and about to support this, and it can be summarized as follows: It always walks as a group and never as a collection of individuals; the walk always takes the time required to support the whole; the faster support the slower. There have been regular occasions when the group has acknowledged this by not getting to the top of a mountain, and they are content to protect the collective aspiration and achievement over any individual personal notion of self.

Recovery groups can also be viewed in terms of the actual impact of the activity and whether process/outcome can be seen as therapeutic to the participating individuals. Thus, for DARE, the actual activity (the outdoor experience) is cathartic: This is apparent even though it is largely informal and unstructured, rather than constructed and controlled in the way of a structured program with an accompanying how-to manual. The psychological benefit of outdoor activity is further reflected in the proliferation of provision aimed at groups as diverse as school children, young offenders, and individuals with learning disabilities. It is also apparent in the growing use of the label "wilderness therapy" and in the existence of an International Adventure Therapy Conference (hosted in 2009 by the British Association of Counseling and Psychotherapy). Equally, although we would defend the particular appropriateness and value of this specific approach, any activity about which you or a group feel passionately could be adopted as the "core" of recovery due to the broader point that it is about involvement, control, acting together, and creating communities of both interest and proximity—in all, promoting a purposeful sense of inclusion.

What this recognizes is that three things—the problems, the solutions, and resources associated with improved futures—do not lie purely in individuals, as consistent with a client-blaming diagnostic approach to drink and drug use, but rather within complex individual, family, and community relationships (White, 2009). This leads to the group redefining notions of what effective treatment or rehabilitation actually is. Recently, a sunny February afternoon stroll down from a hill saw us walking along the banks of a beautiful, hidden mountain lake and discussing (again unconsciously) elements of identification with Mardula's third stage of relapse (Mardula, 1996). Several of us identified a connection between vulnerability, the possible return to old ways, and unfinished work on recovery capital. Once again, the adage, "It's easier to get off than stay off," rings true, an unfortunate fact given the current treatment systems' target-driven preoccupation with enabling folks to get off *at any cost*, even if that is simply onto prescribed medication. This replacement of one addiction with a socially approved alternative offers a form of instant intervention that often completely fails to consider what the individual needs and wants, a source of outcome statistics rather than a means of enabling individuals to sustain long-term sobriety or abstinence (Livingston, 2009). Thus, the walks and the group help folks continue to build both an inner strength and a wider community resource of support. This, in turn, means that the moments of chaos that infiltrate every life and that might have previously resulted in a return to drink and drug use are often successfully navigated, with evidence of improved coping strategies and a general ability to maintain what might be termed a functional life.

This centrality of the role played by community in the recovery process is becoming increasingly understood (White, 2009). Bamber (2009) suggests that community is central to the recovery movement and something that the system cannot produce. DARE is a case in point: a geographical community and a community of interest bound together by a number of collective but disparate elements of identity (outdoor activities, shared histories, mutual self- and joint interests), clearly beyond the ownership or construction of any formal organization or systematic treatment provision. Living in and walking the North Wales mountains has its own specific historical, local, and global context. This sits within and is one of the contextual environments for the integral wider fabric of human psychosocial integration that forms the business of being a human living among other humans in a degree of close proximity (Bamber, 2009). Folks drink and use drugs in their immediate community contexts and will usually have to learn to not drink or use drugs in the same. Ultimately, DARE both creates a community and is of a community: This sense of "local" and the related sense of "us" challenge any broader conception of standardized national delivery or recovery, suggesting as they do the importance of context. The existence of DARE can thus be seen as the unconscious evolution of one of the strategies White (2009) identifies for utilizing communities in supporting recovery, namely the notion of recovery community building including the creation of new social entities, with DARE now being one such entity.

Postchaotic substance use and early recovery is often characterized by individuals struggling with this perception and the reality of being accepted by/identifying with wider sober communities. Frequently, to maintain recovery, they have often had to leave old drinking and drug-using networks behind, thus communities play a crucial role in an individual's sense of belonging. What is required here—what is in fact crucial to continued recovery—is not the complex power-orientated relationships that often result from organizational engagement but simple relationships with nonjudgmental and substance-free peer group(s) (Nordfjaern, Rundmo, & Holi, 2010). As most theories of identity reveal, to be accepted and possess a positive sense of belonging to a community is a basic human need (see, for instance, Tajfel,

Billig, Bundy, & Flament, 1971). It is also commonly a need that has not been fulfilled in people with a history of substance misuse: As we have said, conventional treatment models tend toward enforcement thus implying an offense by an individual against an innocent society, not toward support, which would arguably imply the recognition of a fault on the part of society, carer, or education system toward the individual (Baker, 2010). Obviously, this is simplistic and is in no way intended to undermine the concept of personal responsibility. Recognition of the past does not excuse the individual from responsibility for the future: Simply put, "what has happened has happened, but you are still your only way out of it"—a message that recurs in some form across various counseling models (e.g., Glasser, 1999; Griffin & Tyrrell, 2003; Stewart & Joines, 1987, etc.). Crucially, this does not deny the need for support but makes the case for individual and group empowerment, for working to provide individuals with the mental tool kit to succeed—an essential aspect of recovery arguably at odds with much of our current behaviorist/instructional modeling. Thus, self-help recovery is about the (or a) community *supporting* individuals and is in this context very distinct to any notion of *treating* individuals.

DIFFERENCE

What DARE therefore clearly does—unintentionally, and all the more successfully for that—is creates a sense of identity and belonging, a community of interest within which members have a value and a positive image often denied to them in their everyday life. Again, citing theories of identity and particularly the concept of social construction (e.g., Berger & Luckman, 1967; Gergen, 1999), it can be argued that the traditional treatment cycles have consisted of series of persistent, humiliating discourses that center on blame, drugs (prescription or otherwise), disempowerment, and irresponsibility. As with any form of stigma, the longer this continues, the more self-reinforcing and identity fulfilling the stereotype becomes (e.g., Goffman, 1968). The individual ultimately avoids treatment due to awareness of this situation, or becomes the sum total of these interactions (Radcliffe & Stevens, 2008). Arguably, if the nature of any individuals' daily discourses alters substantially, so does the individual (Burr, 2008; Gergen). This is something that DARE does—or at least starts to do—in that it offers all participants very clear nonblaming/empowering interactions. But then, DARE is not in this sense a treatment model; it did not start by defining an individual in terms of their incompetence ("You're a drug user—you need/want my help . . .") but rather a group of like-minded individuals that is almost incidentally recovery orientated. By assuming participants can do something positive and simple (in this case, just put one foot in front of the other), members begin to rescript each others' discourses, to assume a competence that ultimately takes on solid form. This enabling of positive new futures is at the heart of recovery. Thus, an inclusive and embracing community such as DARE supports and nurtures a positive sense of belonging and achievement.

This is different to a world where the traditional treatment approach offered to this client group tends to consist of a punitive carrot-and-stick approach, medically orientated, intrinsically (and increasingly; Pearson, 1991) linked to the criminal justice system. Studies have shown that this notion of treatment frequently amounts to a bare 10 minutes of structured intervention a week (Best, Day, et al., 2009). From a client's perspective, this amounts to a reinforcement of a sense of low self-worth that arguably explained the substance problem in the first place, and as such, a reinforcement of the key factors that construct our currently understood psychosocial model of substance misuse (e.g., Macleod, 2010). The sense of folks being encouraged and supported in building and maintaining long-term meaningful lives—constructed around a sense of developing personal and community capital—although demonstrably essential (e.g., Nordfjaern et al., 2010), is equally negligible. In this world, if a client is lucky enough to see a hill, then it is at best a day out at the local outdoor pursuits center in a large and partially disinterested group, where the exercise is very much a commissioned process focusing on attendance outcomes. At best, this serves as a day's respite from the hard graft of maintaining the drink or drug use lifestyle; at worst, it serves as a reinforcement of the often-held belief that seeking support through regulation channels is pointless, labeling, and potentially debilitating (e.g., Radcliffe & Stevens, 2008).

As other commentators have noted (e.g., Pennsylvania Drug and Alcohol Coalition, 2009), we are not suggesting that there is no role for clinical treatment. We would, from experience, suggest that elements of this system including substitute prescribing are of value, at least in the short term. For instance, methadone is measurably the most commonly used substitute medication for heroin addiction throughout the world (Bammer, Dobler-Mikola, Fleming, Strang, & Uchtenhagen, 1999), and although it has never lived up to early claims of its efficacy (e.g., Yale Law Journal, 1969), it certainly has a proven role in stabilizing chaotic drug use. Nonetheless, anecdotal evidence points to the efficacy of short-term reducing treatment (although much of the research evidence questions how well this is actioned in reality and suggests an agency tendency to "park" users on a given dose—e.g., Gossop, Marsden, Stewart, & Treacy, 2001). For clinically dominated systems to be more effective, they should be optional not compulsory—a small stepping stone or enabler on the way to the more important business of accessing greater transformational supporting networks and environments, not an end in themselves; they must also include nonprejudicial free access to these broader forms of support. What is crucial here in the distinction between the traditional treatment approach and the recovery group movement is the role of power/control and who owns it. This has been a key aspect in the history of such mutual aid movements as Alcoholics Anonymous and Narcotics Anonymous, which both eschew formal funding and restrict membership exclusively to current and ex-drink and drug users (Kurtz, 1991). While an exclusivity of substance-using membership or an absolute totality of financial independence should not be seen as a prerequisite for a recovery group, the sense of collective shared ownership, participation, and belief almost certainly should.

Recovery, therefore, is about what the individual and community want rather than what any specific agency achieves, where the function of agency should be about the importance of collaboration—helping people to help themselves (e.g., Davis, 2010). This is another of the core principles at the heart of recovery. DARE is a group of individuals helping themselves and helping others to help themselves, a manifestly inherent principle of ownership and inclusion that arguably underlines any successful recovery. This structure offers a balance between the "self" concept and the "other" concept—belonging and participation are very clearly at the center of any recovery group. Best, Day, McCarthy, Darlington, and Pinchbeck (2008) argue that if we look at the traditional treatment approach (in particular the idea of a front-end comprehensive assessment through Maslow's hierarchy of needs model), then the issues of esteem and belonging are often initially missed or unaddressed. This process is usually not revisited or reviewed, and by this omission, fails to support long-term recovery or the building up of personal recovery capital. Instead, clients are often supported by a maintenance[3] - focused model that concentrates on contained harm reduction provision, rather than any journey beyond this point. This statutory approach stops at the point where the journey actually begins and arguably encourages a dependence on both services and substances. In walking together, the group is mutually enabling each other to move on from this point, or (not unusually) without going through this process, meeting some very immediate needs of companionship and belonging while simultaneously creating a space in which longer-term recovery capital building can take place. This sharing of the offer of a change of status means that DARE folks become participants in their own process and journey, "done with" rather than "done to." As simple as this principle is, the result of this sense of inclusion and redefined identity is a predictably strong recovery based on a sense of value and self-worth, reinforced by positive interactions that focus on a previously absent notion of future.

The efficacy of this approach and of the interactions and process framed by DARE is clearly demonstrable through the usual process of outcomes. At a simple and measurable level, members of the group can regularly be seen progressing from chaos to stability and eventually into some form of broader societal engagement. This final stage typically consists of what in other circumstances might be termed agency standard outcomes—employment, volunteering, and education allied to long-term abstinence. At the current time, there are past and present DARE members working in support roles within local organizations, studying for qualifications in carpentry, counseling, and literacy, volunteering in local charity shops, helping to run the harm reduction service, and supporting the Youth Offending Team. Beneficially (and predictably), there are also a number of participants studying for outdoor qualifications, volunteering with outdoor education-directed employers, and pursuing broader personal interests such as climbing, caving, and canoeing.

Allied to this are a wide range of so-called soft outcomes, those vital personal changes to thinking, perception, and ability that stem primarily from the process of interaction and action we have already detailed. These are notoriously complicated to measure (e.g., Dewson, Eccles, Tackey, & Jackson, 2000) and frequently undervalued. They are, however, also at the core of recovery and arguably more important than the hard outcomes we have detailed above: Ultimately, an increase in self-esteem and mindfulness will lead almost automatically to one or more of these other life-changing roles/activities in the fullness of time. Lastly, there has been a significant "knock-on" effect in terms of folks unofficially mentoring each other, engaging as volunteer mentors in the broader substance misuse field, and (slowly but surely) contributing to a rewriting of individual and agency expectations by their actions and progress.

So, we have a self-owned group that creates a sense of belonging to a community and a belief in the self, through which people are able to work on building aspects of their wider positive sober lifestyle. Sobriety here is not that relationship with the substance but the living of a life that has some internally self-rewarding nondestructive qualities—one that enhances rather than damages. The distinction is important to DARE and the wider politics of recovery and knowledge; this is not about removing all risk taking and reducing the individual to a daytime telly couch potato who does not drink but also does not do. We see risk taking as an essential element of the process of transformational growth, both for the individual and the group. Indeed, supporting risk taking is also an acknowledgement that for some, drink and drug use performs a function in terms of taking risks and stepping outside of perceived passive norms—creating excitement and purpose where there is otherwise boredom and drift. Risk taking is further integral to successful recovery in that individuals have to take huge risks in terms of the loss of friendships, networks, and established identities associated with change. This rewriting of a personal life script away from that of the user and toward that of the socially engaged individual is an enormous change that most so-called "functional" folks are never forced to undergo or even contemplate.

Thus, DARE also provides a space and opportunity that is in part an antidote to the risk-averse nature and provision of the mainstream world. The notion of the commissioned walking group would probably exclude those on a prescription, those who are less than so many weeks into residential rehabilitation, or those suffering from anxiety/depression/any other condition that can be vaguely (but often prejudicially) defined as a mental health disorder. For DARE, no such limitations exist: The philosophy of belief in the possibility/probability of inclusivity and achievement override such considerations. Thus, the group will delay the start of its walks until 9:00 am, waiting for the local chemist to open to dispense medication that the area service provider decrees can only be given to such "high-risk" clients on a daily basis. The memory of sheltering in a snowy gully near the summit of Moel Siabod,[4] while a member of the group 2 weeks into detoxification was supported to eat chocolate, get warm, and recover, sits well in many folks' minds. In this instance, the group member would almost certainly never have gotten there (and probably would not have been allowed to try) in any other support system or context; in our story, he and the group as a whole still climbed a mountain that day. It is worth noting that this particular client went on to develop an interest in walking, climbing, and photography, the latter interest now being pursued at college—a journey that certainly owes something to his involvement with the group.

Much of this is, of course, in part due to the refusal of the group to be "professionalized," bound up with the restrictive red tape of becoming an "intervention" or a "project." Attempts by a local service provider a couple of years ago to include the group as a "client activity" to which individuals could be referred were resisted by the simple means of ignoring them when "no" proved to be the wrong answer. That said, although the group does take risks others would not, these are not outrageous risks and are not taken without thought and the resource of a preexisting skill base. The group has had access to some mountaineering expertise ever since that initial conversation between Adam and Brian, and we would emphasize that this common-sense approach is vital to the structure, a part of what defines it, and why it functions. In 5 years of consistent activity, there have been no incidents beyond exhaustion and blisters; consequently, the group does not find itself externally pressured by the oppressive regimes of health and safety that dominate a risk-averse society. As we have said and unpopular as this belief may be, *taking risks promotes growth*: Ask any climber, anyone who has made a major career move, returned to education or—more importantly in our context—taken the massive step of deciding to be substance free after years of living a soap bubble existence. Allied to this is the recognized fact that we learn well in the margins of discomfort and when stretched; we owe it to ourselves and others to allow this to occur, a concept demonstrated by numerous teaching and training models (e.g., Rohnke, 2002).

Genuine inclusivity, the notion of things being initially a little more complex but ultimately more rewarding, is thus at the heart of DARE and recovery group activity. Our understanding of this process, of recovery groups in general, and the specific concept of going the extra mile, despite this not being a designed research project, can nonetheless be informed by our interpretation of the principles of participant action research design (Humphries,

2008). This reflects a collective authorial desire to collate and encapsulate an evidence base in support of the recovery format, both as a product in its own right but also as an alternative to the standardized, controlled approaches of established pharmacological and behavioral responses to substance use. In so doing, we would cite a number of specific points from Whitmore and McGee's principles of action research (2001):

- nonintrusive collaboration (including ownership of the project by the group);
- mutual trust and genuine respect; solidarity (all humanity is connected by a common journey and shared destiny);
- mutuality and equality (everyone's interests are important);
- a focus on process (informal interaction that goes beyond a detached working relationship and respects others' cultures); and
- language as an expression of culture and power.

All of these principles could equally be a part of—and clearly resonate with—our definitions and principles of recovery. Both DARE (which is not a research project) and this article (which is not a research article *per se*) offer us research understanding. These principles are echoed not only in the empowering nature of action research but in core principles of recovery, echoed in this article, journal, and beyond. We might even reasonably ponder whether the whole recovery movement is a mammoth participant action research process in development. In this, then, we have more of the complex power and knowledge issues that impact on the recovery movement and its ability to be legitimately accepted as more than a sideshow to the existing mainstream.

CONCLUSIONS

In drawing these themes together and seeking some form of emergent meaning, we are left with a number of conclusions. DARE is, by our terminological process, a recovery group, at once distinct in itself and representative of other such organizations (or nonorganizations, which is perhaps the point). This role links it inextricably to numerous considerations of power and knowledge and introduces a number of attendant political considerations that are seemingly inescapable in this arena. Some useful reframing of recent key North American work (Alistair, 2010) suggests 12 principles of recovery, which we can again see at work in DARE and which can be usefully added to the "group" part of this definition. The group itself is thus an *honest, aware, nonprescriptive, participative, transformational, antioppressive, self-directed, empowering, opportunistic group of peers and individuals, operating within the community in which they live* (Alistair, 2010). In our earlier pen portrait, we described a group that openly discusses its own direction among its members. Recently, the group has begun to explore mines, walk coastal footpaths, and go rock climbing. This continual evolution from its starting point is an ongoing consequence of reflective chat huddled with butties[5] and a flask.[6] The group chose (and chooses) to listen to those who wanted to go out but did not necessarily see themselves making the big mountains, and as such, evolved in a manner to accommodate all aspirations. As Clark (2010) identifies, this collective, inclusive, integrative, and steadily evolving collection of attributes forms a broad summation of the principles and approaches described in the seminal white paper published by the Recovery-Oriented Systems of Care Subcommittee of the Drug and Alcohol Coalition in Pennsylvania (Pennsylvania Drug and Alcohol Coalition, 2009).

Additionally and interestingly, this article identifies four types of social support: *informal, instrumental, emotional,* and *affiliational,* which it considers to be core to recovery-orientated systems. We hope that in writing this tale, these four types of support have become evident as intrinsic to the working processes of DARE. Thus, folks learn to read maps, use compasses, plan treks, tie ropes, take measured risks, and keep safe, a representative form of *informal support*. By dint of mountainous geography, North Wales is a dispersed community with limited public transport, and as such, most walks are preceded by a complex set of lift-sharing arrangements. Most folks who walk the first time have neither the appropriate footwear nor clothing and are lent such out of the group pool or by other members. In both of these examples, we can see the *instrumental support*, the practical support folks receive to enable them to participate. The group only ever goes as fast as its slowest member, displaying the empathy and concern consistent with *emotional support* for others. The intrinsic nature of this support, however, goes much deeper: The walks can be characterized as 10 or 12 people often astride in pairs or threes "chewing the cud," reviewing each others' lives and recovery, and offering a warm ear and fresh encouragement. This sense of being with others and participating in peer problem solving is not simply typical of emotional support but also of informally facilitated group and individual therapy. Finally, folks feel as though they belong to a group, both in the day as they physically cohabit a space among the recreational walking communities and environments and in the wider community—as such, DARE also provides *affiliational* support.

In summation, we entrust that the tale offered here meets the defining principles of what is and is not recovery as laid out by White (2007) and that it is a celebration of recovery and its diversity, not a questioning of its existence (Best, Groshkova, McCartney, Bamber, & Livingston, 2009). Furthermore, we hope that DARE and the tale as told captures the essential nature and elements of the recovery experience (peer-orientated transformational support), is inclusive in its diversity (open to all and without the stifling client–worker boundaries), is distinctly identifiable (is a monthly reality in the mountains and community of North Wales), is clearly measurable, and has sought to offer an acceptable and interesting account. Above all else, we believe that DARE appears as a typical example of the small nonstatutory sector peer-led organization and as such adheres to Wardle's (2009) aspiration that we put people first. Without the hindrance of commissioners, paperwork, and preoccupations with professional allegiances, DARE has been able to do what matters most: provide a responsive and caring space to accommodate individual personal recovery journeys. As it is also essentially of the mountains and in the mountains, DARE is further evidence of the increasing diversification of mutual aid groups and their philosophical orientation (White, 2009). It is thus a grassroots response to unmet needs (Bamber, 2009), gasping for fresh air amongst the maelstrom of the rigidly imposed, current but seemingly ever-changing, statutory treatment systems.

The strength of any narrative lies in its ability to convince, in the skill of making the reader close their eyes and imagine themselves as a participant, and—in our story—in the gentle determination to affect belief and change. Next Saturday, a group of walkers will meet in the car park below a mountain known as Cadair Idris. The group will be made up of people who began this journey several years ago, new faces who we have yet to meet and—somewhere among them—the authors of this article. This trip has involved a little more planning and a little more sharing than usual: Every participant needs a sleeping bag, warm clothes, food, and a torch. Cadair Idris is a craggy summit, a pleasant seat some thousand feet above a mountain lake in the day time—a dark and slightly intimidating rocky bulk seemingly much further removed from the comforts of so-called civilization by night. Local legend has it that anyone who sleeps on the summit will come down as either a madman or a poet on the following day, a transformation that may have interesting consequences for the future of DARE and—who knows?—this movement as a whole. Recovery, anyone? First mountain on your left, turn right at the stile and keep going … mind the sheep droppings along the way, but if you follow the path, good things can be found round the corner. You might even enjoy the journey in the end.

NOTES

1. Names are fictitious for anonymity and ease of telling the tale.

2. This article has not chosen to engage in a detailed discourse on the use of the term "recovery" (e.g., 12 step or not, abstinent or not). We acknowledge for many who walk in the hills for the first time that this discovery of something new (mountain walking) is possibly a more appropriate term than recovery. But we are comfortable enough with a notion of recovery as folks accessing a less damaging and more rewarding life.

3. Maintenance is both a narrow reference to long-term prescribing programs and the notion of service provision interested in retaining clients within its objectives rather than moving beyond the commissioned treatment context. DARE is open to all and does not hold any membership criteria based on relation to current consumption or not of substance, whether legal, prescribed, illicit, or illegal.

4. Moel is Welsh for "mountain." Moel Siabod is a 2,861-foot (872 meters) mountain near the village of Capel Curig in Snowdonia.

5. Butties is a colloquial term for sandwiches.
6. Flask, as in Thermos Flask or Vacuum Flask, is a container for transporting hot drinks.

REFERENCES

Alistair. (2010). Routes to recovery. *Wired in to Recovery*. [Web Blog]. Retrieved from http://wiredin.org.uk/member/blog/747/entry/6945/routes-to-recovery

Baker, M. (2010). Social exclusion—an addictive context. *The Psychologist, 23*(7), 568–570.

Bamber, S. (2009, October). *Rethinking 'community': Addiction, recovery, and globalization*. Paper presented at the 12th International European Working Group on Drugs-Oriented Research Symposium, University of Stirling, Stirling, Scotland.

Bamber, S. (2010). Recovery glossary. *The art of life itself*. Retrieved from http://www.theartoflifeitself.org/recovery-glossary/mutual-aid-groups

Bammer, G., Dobler-Mikola, A., Fleming, P., Strang, J., & Uchtenhagen, A. (1999). The heroin-prescribing debate: Integrating science and politics. *Science, 284*(5418), 1277–1278.

Becker, H. (1963). *Outsiders: Studies in the sociology of deviance*. New York, NY: Free Press.

Berger, P., & Luckman, T. (1967). *The social construction of reality*. Hammondsworth, UK: Penguin.

Best, D., Day, E., McCarthy, T., Darlington, I., & Pinchbeck, K. (2008). The hierarchy of needs and care planning in addiction services: What Maslow can tell us about addressing competing priorities. *Addiction Research and Theory, 16*(4), 305–307.

Best, D., Day, E., Morgan, B., Oza, T., Copello, A., & Gossop, M. (2009). What treatment means in practice: An analysis of the delivery of evidence-based interventions in criminal justice drug treatment services in Birmingham, England. *Addiction Research and Theory, 17*(6), 678–687.

Best, D., Groshkova, T., McCartney, D., Bamber, S., & Livingston, W. (2009). The politics of hope. *Druglink, 24*(6), 20–21.

Bradbury, H., & Reason, P. (2003). Action research: An opportunity for revitalizing research purpose and practices. *Qualitative Social Work, 2*(2), 155–175.

Burr, V. (2008). *Social constructionism*. London, UK: Routledge.

Clark. (2010). Guiding principles of recovery: From Pennsylvania. *Wired in to recovery*, Retrieved from http://wiredin.org.uk/community/blog/entry/7439/guiding-principles-of-recovery-from-pennsylvania

Clayton, R., & Turnbull, R. (2003). *The Welsh three-thousand-foot challenges*. Hoddlesdon, UK: Greystone.

Daily Mail. (2010). *'Drug users given' search results*. Retrieved from http://www.dailymail.co.uk/home/search.html?searchPhrase=drug+users+given

Davis, F. (2010). Can we sustain the 'magic'? *The Psychologist, 23*(1), 32–33.

Dewson, S., Eccles, J., Tackey, N. D., & Jackson, A. (2000). *Measuring soft outcomes and distance travelled: A review of current practice*. Runcorn, Cheshire, UK: ESF & DWP.

Douglas, T. (1993). *A theory of group work practice*. Basingstoke, UK: Palgrave Macmillan.

Gergen, K. (1999). *An invitation to social construction*. London, UK: Sage.

Glasser, W. (1999). *Choice theory*. New York, NY: Harper Perennial.

Goffman, E. (1968). *Stigma: Notes on the management of spoiled identity*. Harmondsworth, UK: Penguin.

Gossop, M., Marsden, J., Stewart, D., & Treacy, S. (2001). Outcomes after methadone maintenance and methadone reduction treatment: Two-year follow-up results from the National Treatment and Outcome Research Study. *Drug and Alcohol Dependence, 62*(3), 255–264.

Griffin, J., & Tyrrell, I. (2003). *Human givens*. Sussex, UK: HG Publishing.

Humphries, B. (2008). *Social work research for social justice*. Basingstoke, UK: Palgrave Macmillan.

Kurtz, E. (1991). *Not-God: A history of Alcoholic Anonymous* (expanded 1st ed.). Center City, MN: Hazleden Pittman Archive Press.

Livingston, W. (2009). Making sense of the mess in my head. *Journal of New Directions in the Study of Alcohol, 33*, 56–70.

Macleod, J. (2010). Drug taking and its psychosocial consequences. In S. Macgregor (Ed.), *Responding to drug misuse: Research and policy priorities in health and social care* (pp. 25–40). London, UK: Routledge.

Mardula, J. (1996). Turning relapse into change. *Alcohol Concern Magazine, 11*(3), 20–21.

McLellan, A. T. (2010, March). Protagonist of choice. *Drink and Drug News*, pp. 6–7.

Nordfjaern, T., Rundmo, T., & Holi, R. (2010). Treatment and rehabilitation as perceived by patients with substance addiction. *Journal of Psychiatric & Mental Health Nursing, 17*(1), 46–64.

Pearson, G. (1991). Drug policy in Britain. *Crime and Justice, 14*, 167–227.

Pennsylvania Drug and Alcohol Coalition. (2009). *Recovery-orientated system of care: A recovery community perspective* [White paper]. Harrisburg, PA: Author.

Radcliffe, P., & Stevens, A. (2008). Are drug treatment services only for 'thieving junkie scumbags'? Drug users and the management of stigmatized identities. *Social Science and Medicine, 67*(7), 1065–1073.

Rohnke, K. (2002). *A small book about large group games*. Dubuque, IA: Kendall Hunt.

The Scottish Government. (2008). *The road to recovery: A new approach to tackling Scotland's drug problem*. Edinburgh, Scotland: Author.

Shaw, M. E. (1976). *Group dynamics: The psychology of small group behavior* (2nd ed.). London, UK: McGraw-Hill.

Stewart, I., & Joines, V. (1987). *TA today*. Nottingham, UK: Lifespace.

Tajfel, H., Billig, M., Bundy, R. P., & Flament, C. (1971). Social categorization and intergroup behavior. *European Journal of Social Psychology, 1*, 149–177.

Wardle, I. (2009). *Recovery and the UK drug treatment system: Key dimensions of change*. Manchester, UK: Lifeline Project.

White, W. L. (2007). Addiction recovery: Its definitions and conceptual boundaries. *Journal of Substance Abuse Treatment, 33*(3), 229–241.

White, W. L. (2009). The mobilization of community resources to support long-term addiction recovery. *Journal of Substance Abuse Treatment, 36*(2), 146–158.

Whitmore, E., & McGee, C. (2001). Six Street Youth Who Could ... In P. Reason & H. Bradbury (Eds.), *The handbook of action research* (pp. 396–402). London, UK; Thousand Oaks, CA: Sage.

Yale Law Journal. (1969). Methadone maintenance for drug addicts. *Yale Law Journal, 78*(7), 1175–1211.

Yin, R. K. (2009). *Case study research: Design and methods* (4th ed.). London, UK: Sage.

Index